# GOOD HEALTH

# THROUGH

# SPECIAL DIETS

by
Hanna Kroeger

"The Road to Health goes through the kitchen, not through the Drugstore."
Dr. Reidlin, M.D.

"In dedication to all courageous crusaders, past and present, who have and continue to emancipate fellow-man, relieve human suffering, and enlighten all who seek the TRUTH for body, mind and spirit.

# TABLE OF CONTENTS

# INTRODUCTION

All human activity begins with food. Without food we would not be born. Without food we could not grow. If we do not eat, we do not act and react to our lives in a proper, intelligent, and progressive manner. We would not join clubs or society. We would not be able to write books or compose symphonies. We would not go to church. We would not have families.

The production and distribution of food is the first concern of any society.

"What people think, say, and do is determined by the type and quality of the food they eat. Humanity's social, political, economic, and religious behavior depends with and is deeply influenced by food. Its production is not only the first concern of any social group, it is the most important one. The quality of human life—mankind's emotional, psychological, and spiritual health—are all dependent on food."

Diet is not fasting. Diet is arranging certain foods to be eaten at specific intervals. Diets are put into effect:

A. To strengthen the body.

B. To eliminate toxins,

C. To resist disease-causing factors,

D. To influence certain diseases favorably,
E. For better performance,
F. To bring into balance that which is out of balance,
G. For spiritual reasons.

# Therapeutic Diets

Therapeutic diets contain many vegetables, fruits, and sprouted grains. Why? Vegetables and fruits are refreshing. They are easily digested. They have more fibers. They carry more natural vitamins and minerals. Vegetables and fruits prevent the splitting of body-bound protein. In a vegetable abundant diet the acid-alkaline balance is easily maintained. Vegetables, fruits, and sprouted grains have more auxins. Auxins are plant growth harmones. They regulate cell growth in plants. They therefore regulate cell rejuvenation that takes place in the body at all times. Auxins are not easily disturbed by heat. Sprouted whole wheat bread can therefore contain many auxins.

Sprouted seeds are rich in enzymes, B-vitamins, hormones, and aromatic substances.

A few decades ago fruit was considered a luxury food, given to children, or perhaps used occasionaly as a dessert. Vegetables were considered a pleasant and colorful addition to heavy dumplings or to meat dishes. But they were considered more a decoration than a food. We have since learned that fruits and vegetables are good for us nutritionally.

However, no one really knew why they improved health.

Fruits and vegetables have trace minerals. These are most important for the body as all biologial functioning takes place under their influence. Fruits and vegetables have vitamins, particularly when eaten raw. Vitamins are essential for the proper chemical balance of our delicate system. These two food groups have a large amount of cellulose, a fiber, which prevents constipation and residue deposits in the entire digestive tract. Fruits and vegetables also contain auxins, as mentioned, a food for cell rejuvenation. They carry aroma, en-

2

zymes, fruit sugar, and small amounts of special oils which lubricate the tendons, bones, joints, and cells in general.

As raw vegetables and fruits can heal severe illnesses, it stands to reason that these are essential, good, and desirable to the healthy individual, to keep well. If we can be healed by them, we can stay healthy with them.

> **Illness starts** when you give out more energy than you take in.

# THE WILL TO LIVE

The will to live is the will to get well. No matter what the verdict is. Faith carried by the will can make you free from afflictions. The will to live will give you the strength to carry out the diets as mentioned in this book. The will to live will give you the strength to change your uncontrolled lifestyle today. Then you will be in harmony with nature and recuperate completely. Remember, you are responsible for you health. For the sake of your loved ones, change to a good diet. If you are sick, your loved ones have to pay the bills. In addition, they must hear your lamentations all the time. That is not fair. Take full responsibility over this body of yours. Quit cigarettes, quit alcohol, quit sugars and pastries and soft drinks and all that man-made stuff and get on the road to Health, Happiness and Responsible Living, **today**.

Of 100 people, 90 complain of being tired, run down, sleepy, cranky, and exhausted. Out of 100, ninety will ask for more energy.

The importance of proper diet for good health, has been greatly lost in modern time. Among more primitive societies, the basic facts of food were well recognized and used. Finally nutrition, "the youngest branch of science," is making headlines in newspapers and on newsstands. Suddenly people recognize the value of good nutrition. Eagerly they throw out the old system of T.V. dinners and man made food; and, unfortunately also some good nutrition. In any case something is done, good for all of us.

3

# ARTERIOSCLEROSIS
## (Hardening of the Arteries)

When hardening of the arteries sets in, we have to adjust our lifestyle.

No coffee, no alcohol, no potato chips, no heavy cakes or heavy, fatty meals. When arising, exercises, swinging of legs and arms should be considered, so you have to get up 10 minutes earlier.

No heavy lifting no continuous bending (no snow shoveling). At night the stomach should never be overloaded. Cut down on salt and if at all possible, adhere to a meager diet. Don't feel sorry for yourself. Money should not be spent on items which harm the body, the **Temple** of the **Spirit**.

On arising: 7 ounces warm water with a squeeze of lemon to bring the bile to flow.

Breakfast: Fruit and cereal.

Midmorning: Fresh fruit

Noon: Soup with vegetables, barley or millet or rice, vegetables, salads, fish, chicken, turkey or nut dishes of your choice.

Midafternoon: Peppermint or other herb tea, yoghurt and whole wheat bread with butter.

4

Supper: Raw vegetable plate and cooked vegetables as tomatoes, green beans, green peas, cauliflower, broccoli, whole wheat —better rye bread with butter, herb teas, cereal coffee, kefir, yoghurt.

Before each meal take 3 times daily:

> 2 tablets hawthorn berries
> 1 capsule potassium chloride
>    with silica
> 2 tbsp. aloe vera gel in apple juice.

This is for one month.
Then go back to your physician for a recheck.

# ARTHRITIS

| Rheumatoid Arthritis | Oster-Arthritis | Gouty Arthritis |
|---|---|---|
| Age 20-45 | Over 50 | Over 35 |
| Onset insidious (slow) | Onset gradual | Onset acute |
| Pain | Pain | Excruciating pain, clear shiny, tiny nodules around joints. |
| Swelling yes | No swelling | Swelling (sudden swelling and goes down!) |
| Stiffness: yes | Stiffness | Stiffness |
| Tub bath | | Tub bath works crystals out only during acute attacks. |
| Illness progressive up and down, but progressive | Progressive | Intermittent attacks no attacks with proper therapy. |
| General unwell appearance | Well-looking | Looks well |
| Muscles: muscle wasting | No muscle wasting | No muscle wasting |
| Nodules: see them | Not see them | Not see them |
| Deformation: yes | Yes | No |
| Responds to diet well | Responds to diet poorly | Responds to diet poorly |
| Big bumps on fingers, hands crippled, recognized by the looks of it, odd shape of fingers Massage with Tex's Liniment | Nonsystemic disease by degeneration of cartilage of weight-bearing joints, esp. large joints (spine, sockets) 50% nickle poison Put poppyseed on where it hurts. Tex's Liniment | URic acid, crystal accumulation in the blood stream coming from food, pork, cheese, it comes on suddenly to one part of the body. Almost as many deaths from gouty arthritis as from any other. Give male hormone. |

# Suggested Diet for Arthritics

I. The following foods should be included in your diet:

a) All kinds of raw vegetables (except cabbage), water-cress, chard, mustard greens, kale, carrots, celery, lettuce (leaf of Romaine).

These may be eaten with gelatin. This should be Knox Gelatine, taken a minimum of 3 times per week, but better daily. Use the Knox Gelatine recipes: the gelatine may also be taken with tomato juice or other juices.*

Certo is the best joint food there is.

b) Black bread (pumpernickle, rye, or whole wheat).

c) Nuts, especially almonds and filberts (raw nuts are better than those roasted and salted).

d) Fish and sea foods, fowl, lamb, wild game, and liver.

e) Vegetable juices, **citrus fruit juices at times when cereal is not eaten.**

f) Berries, except strawberries.

g) Cooked leafy vegetables (except cabbage); pie-plant (salsify); parsnips; potato peelings from the baked potato, but not the bulk of it.

h) Jerusalem artichoke once each week (they are a root).

i) Great deal of watercress and beet tops (these especially help the eliminations).

j) Most fruits may be eaten, preferably fresh.

II. The following foods should be avoided:

a) These fruits: bananas, strawberries, tomatoes.

b) These vegetables: cabbage, starchy foods.

c) No fried foods; no fats; no pork of any kind, including bacon.

d) No beef, no veal.

e) No malt drinks; no carbonated water (i.e., any soft drinks).

f) No alcohol or spices or other stimulants.

7

# ARTHRITIS

Arthritis is the disease of stress and bottled up negative vibrations. Don't try to reform others, find yourself, reconstruct your subconscious thought, don't lay idle, understand, be patient and loving.

The most outstanding food items conducive to good health for an arthritic are:

| Raw | Cooked |
|---|---|
| Alfalfa seed and sprouted | Turnip greens |
| Clover seed and sprouted | Collared greens |
| Bell pepper | Cauliflower |
| Cauliflower | Broccoli |
| Broccoli | Carrot |
| Parsley | Squash |
| Romaine lettuce | Asparagus |
| Boston lettuce | |
| Papaya | |
| Carrot | |
| Onion | |
| Apple | |

followed by: Tomato, Cucumber, Spinach, Celery, Melon, all fresh Berries, all fresh Fruit, Mushroom, Sweet Potato, Irish Potato. (Fruits alone—Vegetables alone.)

The least desirable foods are: Soft drinks, assorted cookies, White Sugar and White Sugar products, heavy fats, Heavy Syrup, Man-made foods, and foods containing preservatives.

**Poison to an arthritic are:** aluminum, refined food, red meat, sugar, fried food, milk.


# FOR ARTHRITIS

In Germany you are put on a low carbohydrate vegetarian diet. You are sent to a resort. Psychologists try to find the resentment as causative factor for your illness. The body is massaged with castor oil and wrapped in blankets overnight. Herb teas and compresses are administered. Special diets like

Schrot diet, Waerland, and Bircher-Benner are used and lecithin as well as homeopathic remedies are widely advocated.

For arthritis the Italians mix 8 ounces liquid B complex syrup and four ounces of glycerine. They take 6 teaspoons of this mixture a day. Diluted glycerine dissolves hardened mucous collections.

In England they take six tablets magnesium oxide and ten drops phosphorous compound to counteract calcium deposits. Magnesium oxide removes calcium deposits.

In America we follow Mrs. Adelle Davis' stress formula and Dr. Warmbrand's diet suggestion.

In Turkey they bathe in hot springs and wrap the limbs with comfrey leaves.

Dr. Vogel, M.D., a Swiss physician, writes in his book, **The Nature Doctor:**
Before breakfast drink ½ glass of raw potato.
One hour before midday chew three juniper berries.
After meal swallow three mustard seeds.
Between meals drink plenty of potato water.
And the effected parts cover with healing clay or
cottage cheese. The diet whould be absolutely natural.
Old time remedies used in Europe and in America—time proven, effective, simple, and different:
**Stone and Gout Remedy**
  1 quart apple cider
  1 teaspoon hydrangea root
  Let these stand for twelve hours, bring to a boil, simmer.
  Take ½ cup three times daily.

Here is a marvelous recipe to lubricate joints and make joints supple. A young girl, a flower child, gave it to me. I wish I could show to everyone the lovely drawing she put under the recipe.
  1 teaspoon tumeric
  2 teaspoons almond oil
  2 tablespoons soy milk powder
  1 cup water
  salt and honey to taste.
  Heat this and serve as a lovely hot drink.

## Garlic

Chop garlic and fill 1 dessert spoon. Mix with two times the amount of cheese or peanut butter in a sandwich, a slice of bread.

Use Listerine as a gargle for odor.

Do this for 14 days, not leaving out one day. Pain increases at first, then all at once all is gone.

## Rheuma

Take 12 lemons and 4 grapefruit, cut into pieces rinds and all. Run through food grinder, add 3 pints water, bring to boil. Remove from stove at once. Stir in 1 pint corn syrup, mix well. Strain through cloth and cool.

Next dissolve in 1 pint water:

    4 rounded tablespoons epsom salts

    1 oz. sodium salicylate

When dissolved add to fruit 2 tsp. cream of tartar.

All pulp, fill in gallon jug.

Fill jug with more water until full.

Drink 4-6 oz. every day.

or . . . 2 tablespoons Epsom salts

    2 tablespoons cream of tartar

    Juice of 1 lemon, add to qt. boiling water, let cool

    Drink every morning 1 glass.

or . . . 2 times a day take 12 drops of seawater.

# DIET FOR A
# POORLY FUNCTIONING BLADDER

After one has experienced several times, infections in the bladder, one might tell the same story; pain, dribbling, difficulty with urination and irritation. There is nervousness all over. During and after taking drugs to help you, here is something for your diet.

For two days, eat all the alkaline-ash food listed here. I said alkaline-ash food. This is food which increases the alkalinity of the body fluid. In addition, take ½ teaspoon of baking soda in 6 ounces of water, twice a day. Do this for 2 days.

Then switch over to an acid food diet. See the acid producing foods listed here. Eat them on these days. In additon, take 2 teaspoons of vinegar in a glass of water, two times a day, with your meals. Alternate this diet: 2 days alkaline, 2 days acid, for about three weeks.

The strongest infection does not like to be disturbed in this way. No bacterial residue and stronger bacterial strains can develop under the bouncing effect of the alkaline-acid diet.

## Fruits Alkaline

apples*                     grapes*
apricots*                   grapefruit**

11

bananas*
berries*
cherries*
citron*
currants*
prunes increase acidity

raisins****
tangerines**
melon*
oranges*

## Vegetables Alkaline

almonds**
artichokes*
asparagus**
beans, dried
beans, fresh****
beets**
beet tops*
sprouts*
Brussel sprouts*
cabbage*
tomatoes
turnips
spinach
sauerkraut
squash

carrot**
cauliflower*
celery**
lettuce*
mushrooms**
olives*
oninos**
parsley*
parsnip*
peas, fresh*
peppers
raw potatoes,
    with peeling
radish

*Indicates values

You increase your alkalinity with ½ teaspoon soda in 6 ounces water 2 times daily.

The next 2 days, choose only acid foods.

## Acid Foods are

bran**
bread, rye***
cereals**
corn**

rice*
squash*
sugar***
tapioca*

### Starches

cornstarch*
grains*
molasses*
oatmeal**
pastries*

peanuts**
popcorn*
peeled potatoes*
preserves**
spaghetti**

**Protein**

cheese*      chicken
clams***     oysters****
crabs**      turkey***
eggs*       shrimp***
fish        lentils
meats**         *Indicates values

Increase acidity with vinegar water.

By throwing the body juices back and forth, alkaline-acid, the infections will leave for good.

# BLOOD PRESSURE — HIGH

3 oranges
2 lemons

Cut into pieces. Boil in one quart of water for 15 minutes.
Then add 2 tbsp. of honey. Boil another 10 minutes.
Strain and drink six ounces 3 times daily, before meals. (not
 for diabetics)
Oftentimes the kidney diet does miracles for the high blood pressure sufferer.

13

# BLOOD CLEANSER

Put 2 heaping tablespoons of flaxseed in 3 pints of water and boil for 30 minutes. Strain. This will make 1 quart of flaxseed tea. To 1 pint of flaxseed tea, add:

>8 ounces of fruit juice.
>8 ounces carrot juice.

Drink this during the day. Eat fresh fruit in the morning and eat salad and vegetables at noon. Eat yoghurt, buttermilk, rice and vegetables at night. Do this for a few days. You will feel like a bird.

# LOW BLOOD SUGAR DRINKS

1 quart low fat milk
1-2 tbsp. protein concentrate (egg and milk)
2 tsp. protein powder
2 tsp. wheat germ oil (burns slowly, sustains)
2 tbsp. lecithin granules
1 tsp. Tupelo honey
1 or 2 raw egg yolks

Combine with fresh fruit, such as berries, vanilla flavor, and melon, and drink only 2 to 3 ounces at a time, depending on body weight.

# BETTER NUTRITION FOR BRAIN

Knowing that "with the mind we serve the Law of God," this chapter with emphasis on Mental Health for Children is being contributed by Marie Altmann Le Doux, author and publisher of the Play 'N Talk Phonics Program.

Marie Le Doux's efforts in the field of nutrition, especially mental health, have earned for her an Honorary Fellowship in the International Academy of Preventive Medicine.

The BRAIN, an Organ—The MIND, the Intangible You—deserves special consideration. Good Health through one's diet is a direct correlation to good mental health and ability, since a sound mind cannot dwell in a sick and depleted body.

Today's student who figuratively cuts his teeth on TV is programmed for rapid-fire, entertaining teaching. Most teachers are not equipped to match this method. In the absence of such provocative teaching, he withdraws.

Electro-magnetic energy that transpires between the teacher and student brings best results, but it requires optimum health and intelligence on the part of both for success.

Enthusiam, defined: en — in, theos — God, or God within,

15

can only flow from a healthy, peaceful body, not one frought with emotional trauma. An attempt to train a mind that is nutritionally bankrupt, born of parents caught up in the whirlwind of modern scientific man-made foods—pre and post-natally, is sheer folly.

Just as totally healthful foods can only be produced on a naturally fertile soil from seeds that have not been hybridized, there must also be a climate for learning, plus a careful and highly select curriculum for academic success. Knowing that most children now represent the THIRD GENERATION, long removed from the soil, be it farm or back-yard garden, where foods were harvested and eaten immediately, special attention should be given to their DIETS.

Rapid-depletion of vitamin and mineral content resulting from warehousing of under-ripe raw foods, often grown on dead soil, plus transportation and super market exposure, results in such a tremendous loss that supplementation is generally required for optimum health from the cradle to the senior citizen level.

World War II not only undermined the stability of the home by taking the mother out to the factory or office, but it also established those chemical giants who've made a substantial inroad into our dietary format with cleverly appealing advertising for the unsuspecting individual.

Since Dr. N. W. Walker, the eminent scientist and nutritionist, after reviewing our work, devoted a whole chapter to "Play N Talk," in his "Raw Fresh Juice" book (1967), a whole new vista has unfolded for me.

In direct contact with many parents searching for help to overcome their children's reading and spelling problems, it was possible to share pertinent nutritional data, which helped overcome the child's short attention span, poor memory and often hyperactivity. Demands for outlines of supplementation and suggested diet to replace JUNK FOODS, resulted in the release of a 6-page Bulletin,% Nutrition vs Medication for Children with Learning Disabilities. It is by no means confined to the LD area, however. %[Actural case histories

16

are set forth listing vitamin-mineral supplementation, with modifications on entering puberty. And the interview with Dr. Allan Cott, author of "Orthomolecular Approach to Learning Disabilities." High potency B-Complex, plus added $B_3$Niacin (amide) and $B_6$Pryrodoxine are included.]

Since the minerals are the metronome of the body, literally beating out the tune to which the cells must dance, it is important that they be given special consideration. Of the 50 states, over 30 are depleted in the trace mineral ZINC. More and more is being written about this important mineral. It is usually found in abundance when testing the highly intelligent achieving student. It is also regarded as very important in proper development of male reproductive systems, and as a health measure to protect the prostate in the adult male.

Diets eliminating chemicals, both colorings and flavorings, are helpful, but they are not sufficient by themsellves. Eliminating fake-foods and soft drinks without specific helps is like pulling a few bricks out of the corner of a building without replacing them with a better support. The depleted physical and nervous systems result in a state of havoc when it comes to learning. Attention spans, the ability to take instructions and process them, good study habits, a keen memory and the composure to ultimately market the sum total of education require a solid foundation, not based on the HYPE from caffeine, sugar (the robber and thief) nor salted snacks, all of which undermine rather than build.

The BRAIN is a voracious consumer. It is reported that it consumes up to 25% and sometimes more of the body's energy flow as glycogen is released from the liver. An interesting graph was prepared by "LET'S LIVE MAGAZINE" several years ago, showing a direct correlation between JUNK FOODS, plus SUGAR and SALT, with a corresponding decline in grades for students in secondary education. Conversely, diets omitting such items reflected students who were very high achievers!

FOOD is too expensive to waste money on FAKE STUFF.

17

Cooking from "scratch," rather than using chemicalized prepared mixes, is less costly from a monetary and even more so from a hazard to health standpoint.

In the early 70's, I had occasion to be a house guest in Michigan after the parents had successfully used the Play N Talk phonics program to teach their daughter, age 11—Grade IV, to read, in spite of her having been classified as so learning disabled that she would never read. While there, I noticed that this child was a "picky" eater at the table; but a high consumer of cookies and candy between meals. I confronted her mother with this and the possible tragedy that could ensue. Her loving parents helped this little girl change her nutritional intake, and as she went into puberty escaping the proverbial complexion problem among her peers, she has grown into a ravishingly beautiful, self-confident young lady, now completing a very demanding college program.

In September of 1978, a Houston, Texas mother, having learned of my work through Dr. Walker's "Fresh Raw Juice Book," telephone me. Her little girl, age 7½, Grade II, learning disabled, though attending a Learning Center, was very weak in her finer motor skills, not being able to thrust the tongue to the corners of her mouth, though she could project it directly forward. In our chat, I told her of the book "Proven Remedies" by Oliver (1949), as it related to backward children, and the remedies which brought such profound results.

The mother promptly obtained the dulse and eyebright (referred to in the book by Oliver) and made them a part of Erica's diet. Supplementation with these fine herbs abundant in trace minerals, along with our Play N Talk* structured phonics courses, resulted in this child gaining "four years of skills in one semester" as evaluated by the Learning Center. *explained at the end of chapter).

Unable to provide the "one to one" continual sharing of this information, with our inspired work being concentrated in the field of stemming the "tide of illiteracy" I asked Hanna Kroeger to formulate herbs that could be easily available to

18

parents through local health food stores, and if not, directly through her. She measured the potential of these herbs and prayerfully made the combination. Being a capable herbalist, she added Gotu Kola, which further enhances the release of glutamic acid (one of the non-essential amino acids) to the learning center of the brain.

Hanna Kroeger refers to it as **The Cerebral Tonic.** It is designed to feed that part of the brain which converts visualization to comprehension to speech expression. It is a herbal formula consisting of: Gotu Kola, Dulse, and Eyebright. This formula is known to release L-Glutamine (an amino acid) into the brain tissue. L-Glutamine enhances the ability to remember. She called me for a name for it, and we settled for RQ—READ QUICK,—what an inspiration! If IQ means intelligence quotient, surely READ QUICK is right on target. It is SUPER—it is for ALL AGES, improves memory, reduces brain fatigue. What a blessing.

KICKING THE COLA HABIT, often established when the child is just a toddler, is not easy, since caffeine and sugar are highly addictive. Over-sugaring prepares for junior alcoholism, sugars being either fruit or grain alcohol, and as tolerance develops, the craving increases. It takes more to satisfy. Caffeine and sugar viciously interfere with learning, often contributing to Low Blood Sugar problems, which are not discovered since the hyperactive child is medicated rather than the source of his problem unveiled, and he is being patterned for possible future drug abuse.

For Good Recipes see Special Section.

# CLAY DIET

Clay for healing has been used since mankind existed. Even the Bible tells us how Jesus took clay for healing the sick and as an instrument of His Divine power.

How does volcanic ash work? According to leading experts on geology, volcanic ash has one of the world's smallest molecules. These molecules are shaped like calling cards. The two broad surfaces have a negative electrical attraction, while the edges are positive. Therefore, volcanic ash can pick up many times its own weight of positive charged ions. Certain toxins and bacteria found at times in the body and in the alimentary tract in particular are of positive charge. Volcanic ash absorbs or neutralizes such intruders, and in this way volcanic ash aids in the detoxification of the alimentary canal. It took an ingenious American man to realize these facts and to have the foresight to bring a product to the market which everyone can use in confidence and to full benefit. Mr. Irons took volcanic ash and emulsified it in a truly ingenious way. His product stays in suspension and does not settle to the bottom of the bottle.

Whenever the problem of health is partially or totally due to a toxic, overloaded alimentary tract, this scientific and therefore very effective fast on volcanic ash should be considered. Here it is:

Take 2 to 3 tbsp. of liquid bentonite in one glass water.

Take 1 heaping tsp. of detox or psyllium seed or intestinal cleanser (a bulk-making item) in one glass unsweetened juice.

Drink more fluids, like herb tea or water, after that, so you have a total fluid intake of 16 ounces.

Do this five times a day: at 7 a.m., 10 a.m., 1 p.m., 4 p.m., and 7 p.m. At 9 p.m. take an enema to eliminate all the waste from the colon so you may sleep soundly. On the fourth or fifth day you will lose beside long ropes of waste, black matter, which is the sign that you may start adding food to your diet, such as some raw and steamed vegetables, and raw and steamed fruit. Discontinue clay after the seventh day, re-establish friendly bacteria with acidophilus or yoghurt, and go on a good natural diet.

This fast is modern. It is without hunger pangs. It is effective and helpful.

# COLDS

Make an onion soup.

    Take ½ cup white onions

       ½ cup red onions

Saute onions in a little butter, and add:

       1½ cups tomato juice

       1 tsp. boneset — optional

       1 tsp. coltsfoot— optional

Simmer for 5 minutes and et it hot.

In many cases of colds when the PH has slipped the Vitamin C cannot be absorbed. The onion soup changes the PH so the Vitamin C can work again.

Very important to know.

(See Fever Diets)

# CLEANSING
## (Seneca Indian) Cleansing Diet

This diet was contributed by the Seneca Indians.

First day: Eat only fruit and all you want. Try apples, berries, watermelon, pears, peaches, cherries, whole citrus fruits, and so forth. No bananas.

Second day: Drink all the herb teas you want, such as raspberry, hyssop, chamomile, or peppermint. You may sweeten the tea slightly with honey or maple sugar.

Third day: Eat all vegetables you want. Have them raw, steamed, or both.

Fourth day: Make a big pot of vegetable broth by boiling cauliflower, cabbage, onion, green pepper, parsley, or whatever you have available. Season with sea salt or vegetable broth cubes. Drink only this rich mineral broth all day long.

This diet has the following effect. The first day the colon is cleansed (your waste paper basket). The second day you release toxins, salt, and excessive calcium deposits in the muscles, tissue and organs. The third day the digestive tract is supplied with healthful, mineral rich bulk. On the fourth day the blood, lymph, and inner organs are mineralized. That makes a lot of sense!

## TISSUE CLEANSING

Make for yourself 6 ounces of fresh orange juice ten times a day. Add 2 ounces of distilled water and drink slowly. Drink a hot tea made from wood sanicle and peppermint 3 times a day, that is, morning, noon and night.

After 2 to 3 days, your skin will be different. The calcium deposits in your body will be lessened due to the lime in the oranges. You may continue the orange juice another 3 days, but eat apples, pears, berries and a few nuts.

# COLON
## Ulcerative Colitis

The cause of ulcerative colitis is unknown. Is it an allergy or an emotional upset? Is it pesticide residue, metallic poisoning, chemical residue, or pollution? In either case, the mucous lining of the colon becomes inflamed until it bleeds.

"Whatever the cause, something inflames the mucous lining of the colon until it bleeds. Ulcers can pit its surface. Small, worm-like stubs—pseudopolys—grow in scattered clumps.

"During an attack of this inflammation (which can last for weeks and then not appear again for years), the colon is useless. It can't absorb water, and it can't stop the rush of liquid feces into the rectum.

"The result of course is diarrhea. In mild ulcerative colitis, the diarrhea is bearable. In severe ulcerative colitis it is not.

"You have to run to the bathroom. Immediately after defecating, you feel the urge to defecate again—and again, until the bathroom turns into a prison. You're weak and sickly. You run a high fever. Your painful abdominal cramps never let up. Anemic from the loss of blood, your only desire is to stay in bed (standing up makes your diarrhea worse).

"In a survey of 84 people with ulcerative colitis, 72 said that during a severe attack social life was impossible because of fear of incontinence, the embarassment of sudden trips to the bathroom and tiredness."

In considering the food intake of these very sick people, we always have to think of the possible allergic reactions to one specific food or combination of foods.

Ask your physician to conduct an allergy test of wheat, oats, barley, rye, corn, milk, milk products, and other items. You will have to learn to avoid the foods to which you are allergic.

Here is a diet without grains or milk products. Add to that which your allergy doctor allows you to have.

On arising: Drink warm chamomile tea without sugar.
Breakfast: Have two soft-boiled eggs with mashed potatoes, ground flaxseed with soy milk, slippery elm drink with soy milk and warm chamomile tea.
Midmorning: Have two raw grated apples.
Lunch: Eat very well done rice or millet; boiled and mashed carrots with butter, when allowed; squash with tamari sauce, ground flaxseed or tahini; soup or any other warm liquid.
Afternoon: Drink warm tea with rice crackers or millet cereal.
Supper: Eat baked potatoes or mashed potatoes with cauliflower or mashed rutabaga; have tofu if wanted; eat squash, carrots and beets.
Bedtime: Enjoy yoghurt made from soy milk; drink chamomile tea.

You have to work closely with your physician. When you graduate to chicken or beef, take only small, small portions to observe the reactions.

# CONSTIPATION

The causes of constipation are many-fold. There can be a paralysis of the alimentary tract due to Polio, arsenic poison or lead poison.

There can be severe obstructions caused by a nest of worms or a tape worm. It could be that the intestines have dropped or there could be a tumor forming.

All above mentioned things are beyond the pages of this booklet and should be helped by a physician, a chiropractor, or a naturopath.

Besides the above mentioned causes for constipation, there are three different conditions of the tract which need 3 completely different diets.

The first one we call **alimentary constipation**
The second            **atomic constipation**
The third              **spastic constipation**

The **alimentary constipation** is most widespread. It is caused by a fiber-low diet and the large intestines become lazy and lacking in peristaltic movement.

This kind responds very well to diet:

On arising: An apple or a glass of fruit juice or six prunes soaked a day before.

Breakfast: Cereal with ½ bran and ½ wheat germ and fresh fruit or berries. Bran is oftentimes too rough and cuts delicate membranes; combined with oil-containing wheat germ it is perfect. Whole wheat bread, cream with water and honey.

or: Eggs with a mixed salad as tomatoes, cucumber, pepper.

or: Pancake made out of whole grains, granola with lots of fruit, whole wheat bread and butter.

Lunch: Large salad and vegetables, protein as meat, chicken, turkey, fish (no rice)

Midafternoon: Kefir or yoghurt.

Supper: Salads, vegetable soup, yoghurt

or: fresh fruit with yoghurt and whole wheat bread.

The **atomic constipation** is the result of the first kind. The colon does not react to a fiber-rich diet any longer. The friendly bacteria in the alimentary tract are weak or wiped out. The colon has to be stimulated by exercises, sport, light massage (do-it-yourself type), and in some cases even electrical-vibration massage is indicated.

Before each meal take a small plate of raw sauerkraut.

You may prepare sauerkraut with apples, green pepper, caraway, or other goodies. A saucer full of sauerkraut is enough.

In general follow the diet for alimentary constipation but add acidophilus to this diet, and much more kefir and yoghurt.

Also soak 2 tsp. flaxseed in juices and drink this 3 times daily. Yu also may grind the flaxseed and add it to your food. It tastes very good and nutty if it is ground fresh.

### General Rules for Relieving Constipation

1. First rule: Always plenty of pure water to drink!

2.  Fresh fruits and vegetables are very important because of roughage. Stewed and dried fruits are also helpful.
3.  Add unprocessed wheat bran and/or unprocessed wheat germ to your daily diet to normalize bowel function.
4.  Brewer's yeast is effective for many.
5.  Avoid excessive milk drinking.
6.  Daily morning or afternoon exercise, Yoga, walking in fresh air, etc.
7.  Go to the bathroom daily at the same time after a meal, relax, read there, stay a while.
8.  Reflex-Massage stimulates the circulation of every gland in the body!
9.  Body-Massage: Natural therapy, improves: Circulation, Digestion, Respiration, Organs of Elimination, Brain and Nervous System (receive greater supply of blood).

### Spastic Constipation

Spastic constipation diet is just the contrary of a cellulose-rich diet. The colon, the whole alimentary tract is in an uproar. Part of the colon closes. Small balls of feces are expelled or a pencil-thick stool sometimes like a ribbon is expelled.

Oftentimes this spastic condition is an allergy to a food (wheat, eggs, milk), or it could be a pesticide residue or heaven knows what.

I had a lady, she had an allergy to her houseplants. A man was allergic to loud noises, a child to the dishwashing compound mother used, and so on. The colon reacts to life's influences.

No. I: More love and understanding.

No. II: Very little bulk.

### Sample menu for Spastic Colitis

Breakfast: 1 tbsp. ground flaxseed
1 dish cooked oatmeal with cream or butter, toast, Zwieback, honey in most cases allowed.

Midmorning: Freshly pressed fruit juice or kefir or yoghurt.

Lunch: Soup made out of rice, barley or oat well done.
Some fowl or fish and vegetables.

Midafternoon: Yoghurt or better, fresh pressed vegetable juice.

Supper: Cottage cheese, 1 soft-boiled egg, rice crackers with butter or menu as at noon.

At Bedtime: 1 tablespoon flaxseed in water, some applesauce if you desire.

## For a Spastic Colon

Rutabaga is the finest food to relax a spastic colon. It also builds up friendly bacteria.

Cut rutabaga in small pieces. Cover with water and bring to boil. Add thickly peeled potatoes (one large handful) and simmer 'til all is done. Mash it or place it into a blender to have a fine mush. Season with butter, salt, nutmeg (optional).

You may add many things as a side dish as green vegetables and finely chopped greens.

# DU PONT DIET

Much talked about is the "Du Pont" Diet. It is really an Eskimo Diet. Very rich in fat, rich in meat proteins and void of all sugars or starches.

It is said to improve:
> Arthritis
> Arterial troubles
> Diabetis
> Heart trouble
> Obesity
> Lack of Vitality, and others.

I have not tried this Diet and I have no experience in its value.

By all means if you want to try it eat plenty of green vegetables with it. Remember the Eskimos always eat the content of stomach and intestines of the caribou and their fish and seal also, that is the secret of their supplementation.

# ELECTRO MAGNETIC ENERGY DIET

W. H. Hay, M.D., believes he has found a method to develop and ensure a healthy digestion. He separates protein meals from carbohydrate meals. It is his opinion that in mixing carbohydrate and protein at the same meal, we end up with intestinal trouble. Gas develops, and worst of all, locked proteins.

Therefore, it is recommended for:

Breakfast: **Protein.**
    a. Eggs or cheese or meat with a vegetable salad.
    b. Hormone cereal and no bread. See recipe.
    c. Bread with cereal with honey and fruit.

Noon: **Have either a protein meal or a carbohydrate meal.**
    a. Protein with salad and green vegetables.
    b. Carbohydrate, i.e. pancake, wheatbread, or noodles.

Don't eat a cheese sandwich or a tuna fish sandwich or a hamburger. Grains and proteins should definitely be separated. This separation of protein and carbohydrate is not directed toward a specific disease, but is rather a lifestyle. Once you have started it, you will never deviate from it. You begin to feel alive, bouyant, healthy and happy.

---

### Electro-Magnetic Energy in Foods

Every living body has an electro-magnetic forcefield. The higher this forcefield, the healthier the body. The lower the forcefield, the more the body needs help to generate this energy and people feel low in energy.

---

The electro-magnetic forcefield, also called "Aura," in esoteric circles, is a protective layer around the body and each organ in particular. A protection against all kinds of intruders, including dark forces.

Every food has an electro-magnetic power. Every food is eager to release its power and ready to increase your energy. However, here comes the astoundingly incredible new and beautiful knowledge on how to combine food, so it can release its electro-magnetic force and feed the protective shield around us.

Vegetables above the ground, combined with grains, release an enormous quantity of energies and the body is able to absorb every bit of it.

Also, vegetables above the ground, combined with protein, become a super-charger.

Vegetables below the ground, combined with protein, release a fair amount of energies, like meat with potatoes and carrots.

Grains with fruit juice build mucous in the stomach and nulligy the energy patterns.

Grains and protein, taken at the same time, nullify the electro-magnetic power completely. (Only rice is an exception. It hinders the flow, but does not nullify it completely.) This means for anyone low in energy:

No bread with eggs.

No bread with sausage or meat.

No bread in meatloaves.

No bread with cheese.

No dinner rolls when meat is served.

For anyone low in energy, no milk with meat. This is a law already mentioned in the Bible. Milk neutralizes the stomach acidity. Meat needs a lot of acidity to be digested. So, meat with milk will sit in the stomach and will decay. Besides, meat and milk do neutralize the electro-magnetic pattern and you have a complete void.

God placed fruit on the trees and vegetables on the ground, so we would not mix them at the same meal. But we do not listen. We eat fruit pies after a vegetable meal. We mix fruit into a vegetable salad. We serve peaches on lettuce and cherry cobblers after a meat-salad sandwich. And then we harp that we do not have energy.

# ENERGY DIET

On Arising: 1 glass distilled water, hot or warm with some lemon juice in it.

Breakfast: Egg and salad or protein (chicken, breakfast steak)

or: Cottage cheese and salad or fruit.

or: Whole wheat bread and cereal.

If you decide on protein, then eat no bread with it; protein and bread or cereal will not release the energy into the cells.

At 10 A.M.: Apple or other fruit, fresh fruit juice Food supplement.

At Noon: Fish and vegetable and salad, rice allowed.

or: Chicken and vegetable and salad, rice allowed.

or: Meat and vegetable and salad.

or: Any other protein with vegetable and salad. Herb tea and food supplement.

Afternoon: Fresh fruit juice.

Supper: Yoghurt and fruit.

or: Mixed salad and vegetable, whole wheat bread, rye bread.

or: Vegetable soup and whole wheat bread, rye bread.

Bedtime: Yoghurt, honey and calcium, if wanted.

# ELECTLRO-MAGNETIC FOOD COMBINATION

## ELECTRO-MAGNETIC FOOD COMBINATION

| 1 | 2 | 3 | 4 | 5a | |
|---|---|---|---|----|---|
| All Sea Food | Spinach | Sweet Milk, raw | Cherries | Lentils | Combine 1 and 2 |
| Whole Eggs | Avocado | Yogurt | Apricots | Beans, dried | |
| Lamb | Watercress | Cream | Peaches | Mushrooms | |
| Beef | Okra | Filberts | Pineapple | Peas, dried | Combine 3 and 4 |
| Potatoes, White | Beets | Tea-(Lemon) | Grapes | Egg Plant | |
| Potatoes, Sweet | Radishes | Gelatin | Plums | Peanuts | |
| Eggs | Parsnips | Bread-Whole grain | All Berries | 5b | Combine 5a with 2 + Corn Rice, Millet Greens above ground. |
| Veal | Salsify | Steel Cut Oats | * * | Tea | |
| Oyster | Lettuce | Cereals | Bananas | Grapefruit | |
| All Fish | Kraut | Corn Meal | Melons | Lemons | |
| Olive Oil | Kohlrabi | Maple Syrup | Molasses | Limes | |
| Rutabagas | Beet tops | Almonds | Brown Sugar | Watermelon | |
| Tomatoes, Fresh | Dandelion | Wheat Germ | Preserves-honey | 5c | 5b by itself |
| Tomatoes, Cooked | Brussels Sprouts | Goats Milk, raw | Raisins | Cooked or canned | |
| Rice | Peppermint | Buttermilk | Dates | Tomatoes | |
| Oils | Broccoli | Cheese-natural | Figs | Spaghetti | Combine 5c with 2 |
| | Green Peas | Butter | Pomegranates | Rice | |
| | Cauliflour | Cottage Cheese | Currants | Corn | |
| | Green Pepper | Millet | Rice, Brown | Millet | Apples and Rice are Universal |
| | Carrots | Rice | | | |
| | Green Corn | Bread | | | |
| | Onions | | | | |
| | Cress | | | | |
| | Green Beans | | | | |
| | Cabbage | | | | |
| | Escarole | | | | |
| | Asparagus | | | | |
| | Pumpkin | | | | |
| | Cucumbers | | | | |
| | Chard | | | | |

# OLD EGYPTIAN SECRET
## To Draw Higher Energies

The following recipe was used by the Egyptians. They claimed the food combinations given below raise the vibratory forces within the body. They gave it to the elderly to give them energy. They claimed that it is strength-building. They recommended it to those who worked with spiritual healing and higher energies. They gave it to the children. They liked it not only for all those properties, but also because it regulates colon activities.

Take 1 cup black figs (dried)
    1 cup dates (dried)

Cut both in small pieces, add plenty of water, about 1 quart, and bring this mixture to a boil. Do this **very slowly.**

When it boils, add yellow corn meal until it is semi-thick (about ½ cup). Add ½ tsp. salt and serve with cream or milk. Hot or cold, it is delicious. This mixture is also good for:

    anemia
    general weakness
    poor elimination
    gas formation
    and, it brings the people with alcoholism
    to their senses.

A 30-year old lady, depressed, unhappy, listless, incoherent, was served this food 3 times daily. It was the greatest miracle, to observe this poor soul coming to life. For 3 days there was no change, and then it was as if a faucet with sparkling water was turned on. The dried up human plant came to life with miraculous results and in service to others.

# FASTING
## FOR SPIRITUAL REASONS

Fasting for spiritual reasons is practiced widely by our precious youth. It is a fad, unfortunately—an ego trip for many to fast senselessly for prolonged periods of time. They go on water, the worst they can do, and over-draw their capacity of fasting to the point of delayed return or even no return.

Please, young people, listen. Do not go on water fasts. Water fasts can flush high toxicity due to fallout and chemical poisons into the blood stream. The responsible way to fasting for spiritual reasons is the following approved method. It is very, very effective.

Take one pound mannukka raisins and soak them in four quarts water, distilled preferred, for 24 hours. Stir frequently and drink 1-1½ quarts of the water in small sips in the morning from 7 a.m. to 11 a.m., or 8 a.m. to noon. For one hour take neither food nor drink, and have lunch consisting of vegetable and salad and fish or eggs or cheese. The supper is your choice of food, but should not be taken later than 6 p.m. Do this for two to four weeks, or as you feel it is necessary. Meditate short periods, five to ten minutes, several times a day. It is not the length, it is the depth that counts for us Westerners.

You may also use 36 ounces of grape juice in the above described manner; however, you have to add six ounces of water to the 36 ounces of grape juice in order for it to work. Why? I don't know. It must be a secret of the electro-magnetic field, which we do not know too much about.

38

# FEVERS

In all fever diseases there should be a fasting period of 2 days. The patient should have plenty of liquids as:
> diluted apple juice
> diluted grape juice
> herb tea with honey
> cherry juice
> fresh orange juice
> lime and lemonade

and herb teas as:
> feverflue
> chamomile
> peppermint
> and others

When patient asks for meals give:
> buttermilk
> kefir
> stewed fruit or
> yoghurt

No sweet milk is allowed

The body needs fluid, Vitamin C-rich fluid. The liver

needs carbohydrates available in the fruit juices, so the cells of the liver will not be damaged by lack of glycogen. On the third day start with:

>fruit and fruit soup
>light vegetables
>toast and some butter
>peas
>carrots
>beets and others

In fever diseases a glycogen enriched liver can more easily cope with the situation than a glycogen poor liver. Therefore, in all fever diseases, diluted fruit juice, honey sweetened tea and such should be offered.

The natural antibiotics are:

| Garlic | Parsley and radish |
| Grapefruit | Willow |
| Chlorophyl | B-pollen extract |

# HIGH-FIBER DIET

One of the reasons that modern man does not eat a high-fiber diet is that we all do not take time to eat. A fiber diet needs chewing and chewing thoroughly. That takes time. Since modern man and especially women take only 10 minutes to eat lunches and 5 minutes for breakfast, mankind has come up with the practical solution to this dilemma. We serve a soft food drink that can be swallowed quickly.

Protein drink for breakfast
Donut and coffee between telephoning
Soft bread and soft cheese for lunch
A small salad for supper with mashed potatoes
and meat
Cakes and cookies on top.
Just not enough fiber!

The principal function of fiber is to normalize the digestive system, allowing efficient elimination of waste products.

Fifty years ago the low fiber diet was started.

Since then the modern man suffers with constipation, diverticular diseases, hemorrhoids, appendicitis, ulcerative colitis, cancer of the bowel.

Modern nutrition has found that when more fiber-rich food is given, the above mentioned diseases rarely exist.

When we think of fiber food, we think of bran. Yes, it is the richest food in fiber. However, it has a drawback. The sharp edges of the bran may injure the already sick colon. Please add wheat germ to your bran. Wheat germ is also high in fiber, but has some health-giving Vitamin E and rich oils in it which lubricate the bran and the danger of bran bulking in the intestines is over.

Raw and cooked vegetables, whole grain breads, fruits and berries, beans and corn all have fiber and will keep a healthy colon doing its best. Once a colon is sick, weakened and diseased, special care and diet have to be taken.

I summarize: Recent findings tell us that fiber "is the important thing."

Formerly, we were told not to use fiber, as it might cause a variety of colon troubles.

Where is the truth?

The truth is the wholeness of food. The carrot has fiber, the whole potato has it, the grains have bran and in this natural fiber are hidden minerals which we will not get if we eat only a part of the wholeness.

Here are physicians' opinions on high-fiber diets:

Dr. Andrew Stanway, a former chief physician at Kings College Hospital in London, England, and a nutrition expert, explains how: "the swift movement of bran through the body means that cancer-causing agents in food have less time to start that process that would cause colon cancer. This fast movement also prevents conditions such as gallstones, stomach ailments, and circulatory problems."

Dr. Siegal ("Dr. Siegal's Natural Fiber Permanent Weight Loss") says his clinics have used it with success on 5,000 patients in the last year. "A high-bran diet with few refined carbohydrates such as that developed by Dr. Siegal will safely take pounds off you and keep them off."

Emanuel Cheraskin, M.D., chairman of the Department of Oral Medicine at the university of Alabama and author of 13

books on the relationship between diet and disease, writes of
the high-fiber diet: "It will help prevent heart disease, colon
cancer, gallstones, stomach ailments, hemorrhoids, and blood
clots."

Bran, a natural food fiber, is tasteless and easy to take.

Mix 3 tablespoons bran and 3 tablespoons raw or
toasted wheat germ.

**"You just add it to any kind of food you want, from soup to
cereals to ground beef."**

# LIVER

## Liver and Gallbladder Rejuvenating Diet

Prepare:
    2 oz. raw (beets and greens) juice — put in
    3 qts. water plus
    2 cups fresh lemon juice
    2 tablespoons tupelo (or other) raw honey
    (Stir water and lemon together — add honey):

| | |
|---|---|
| 7:00 a.m. | 2 glasses apple juice |
| 9:00 a.m. | 2 glasses beet-lemon juice |
| 11:00 a.m. | 2 glasses apple juice |
| 1:00 p.m. | 2 glasses beet-lemon juice |
| 3:00 p.m. | 2 glasses apple juice |
| 5:00 p.m. | 2 glasses beet-lemon juice |
| 7:00 p.m. | 2 glasses apple juice . |
| 9:00 p.m. | 2 glasses beet-lemon juice |

Do this for 2 days, if possible, 3 days. The result is phenomenal!

Take an enema if needed, or if you feel toxic.

## Cleansing Diet for the Liver
## Quick Method

To begin:

The first day on arising, drink 8 ounces of hot water with fresh lemons squeezed into it. From then on, eat whenever hungry, stewed tomatoes and tomato juice. This acts as a cleanser. Drink hot water and lemon or tomato juice whenever you feel like it. The more the better. Do not worry about the following day, because it is the same procedure. It is amazing how hungry you become. So at bedtime of the second day, you will look forward to the following cocktail:

3 ounces olive oil
2 ounces castor oil
3 ounces whipping cream

Drink this before bed when you are ready for sleep and relaxed. You may chew a little piece of lemon afterwards just for taste. It is a lot easier than it sounds. At 3 or 4 a.m., you will be having a nature's call and in all your life, you have not experienced so much dark and ugly smelling waste. The next morning have a breakfast you desire and earned.

Accumulation of toxins in the body may occur due to failure of the detoxification systems: liver, kidney, thyroid, adrenals and colon. Accumulation may also be due to faulty metabolism or toxid matter.

### For a Healthy Liver:

½ quart carrot juice
½ quart goats milk
1 tbsp. molasses per quart

or:

½ tsp. nutmeg in a cup of hot water
Midmorning 1 cup
Midafternoon 1 cup

### Formula for Cleansing Liver and Pancreas:

Soak 1 lb. dried apricots in pineapple juice over night. Next morning blend it and add fresh pineapple pieces and juice so that it becomes thick enough to spoon it. Divide it in four portions and eat if morning, noon, night and bedtime—preferably not eating anything else that day.

**Also for the Liver:** 1 hour after breakfast drink
6 oz. carrot juice.

### Spleen and Liver Cleanser

Ingredients: 2 quarts of Concord grape juice
juice of 6 oranges
juice of 3 lemons

Cut the white of the lemon into small pieces. Boil this in a little water for ten minutes. Add the water to the drink. Then take distilled water and fill the liquid mixture to 1 gallon. This is one day's supply of your food-drink intake. Just two days of this will cleanse your organs, as drano cleanses your water pipes.

### Dr. Reams' Water Drink

Dr. Reams said that "distilled water is a healing water, when you use it right." 3 to 4 ounces of distilled water every ½ hour, all day long will eash out protein, nitrogen and poisons from the tissue. He said that as soon as you take more water, the water will be eliminated quickly through the kidneys and sweat. This is a very good plan for all of us. It will not hurt to do this once in a while, for two days in a row.

### Liver Rejuvenating Recipes

I found the following recipe in an old book used in 1802 by Dr. Selig of Austria. It sounded so good that I tried it and found that it is truly excellent.

Boil: 1 tsp. dandelion root
1 tsp. angelica
1 tsp. wormwood
1 tsp. gentian

Simmer in two cups water and strain.

Add: 2 quarts apple juice and 4 oz. freshly squeezed lemon juice, and drink this in small portions during the day. Do this for 2-3 days and repeat if needed once a month. Take only stewed fruit and apple juice on these days.

Mrs. Fisher had beautiful hands and arms, but large spots of dark pigmentation covered them. These pigmentations grew worse from year to year. When I shared with her the above recipe, she was all for it—and what wonders! The dark circles and "age spots" faded and slowly disappeared.

# GALLBLADDER

In the case of acute infection of the gallbladder, do not give anything to eat. Make a tea of Horsetail, Nettle, Yarrow, Mint and Dandelion. Give at the onset of discomfort, only one tablespoon of tea every ½ hour. In addition, make a milk compress over the gallbladder area. Make the compress cool or warm. Whatever feels best. Once the gallbladder is infected, you have to heal this trouble spot thoroughly. Your physician will help you. And you help him by staying on a strict diet regimen. Here I give you No! No! foods:

## No No Food in Gallbladder Infection

All food that is fried:

| | |
|---|---|
| potato chips | alcohol (any kind) |
| fried hamburgers | pepper |
| fried eggs | spices |
| pancakes | whole milk |
| cakes | whipping cream |
| pork | fat cheese |

The food must be light and wholesome, such as:

| | |
|---|---|
| vegetables | steamed fruit |
| rice, millet, oats | fruit and vegetable juices |

|          |                       |
|----------|-----------------------|
| potatoes | skim milk, soy milk   |
| chicken  | all seasoned with herbs |

On arising: take lemon juice in warm water with a little honey.

### Apple Juice Diet

I have a book from the 17th century in which an old physician from Austria gives his secrets. One of them is the apple juice diet. This diet is greatly used among health-minded people to detoxify liver and gallbladder. Here is one report. "I had a very bad summer. Too much work, too little sleep. I did not take food supplements and had to work under conditions where I had to eat fried food and other No No foods. In the fall it started. Tired, bloated, listless, I caught myself being sarcastic and nasty. One night I had terrible pain over my right shoulder and neck. I am sorry to say my liver quit her job, and the next morning I went on the apple juice diet. The bright green pebbles, the old bile just poured out on the third day, and I was myself again."

Here it is, and I recommend it to everyone very, very highly. Give your liver a rest, a chance, a holiday.

**First Day:**

| | | |
|---------|-------------------|-------------|
| 8 a.m.  | 1 glass   (8 oz.) | Apple Juice |
| 10 a.m. | 2 glasses (16 oz.) | Apple Juice |
| 12 p.m. | 2 glasses (16 oz.) | Apple Juice |
| 2 p.m.  | 2 glasses (16 oz.) | Apple Juice |
| 4 p.m.  | 2 glasses (16 oz.) | Apple Juice |
| 6 p.m.  | 2 glasses (16 oz.) | Apple Juice |

(Juice should be natural, without chemicals)
No food is to be taken this day.

**Second Day:**

Same procedure as for the first day. No food this day either.

At bedtime of second day, take 4 oz. olive oil. You may wash the olive oil down with hot lemon juice or hot apple juice.

Go to bed at once.

As a rule this diet starts to work around 4 a.m. In the fecal matter you will find little green pebbles. They may be the size of a pin head or they may be as big as a bird egg. Many times it all looks like green mud.

In any case, the old stagnant bile becomes dissolved and liquefied through the malic acid of the apple juice. The oil moves the whole mess.

Dr. Adolphus Hohensee had been using this diet on thousands of his students all over America. In Europe it is practiced in health spas and hospitals with equal results. It re-establishes the normal function of the liver. This diet "frees the liver-gallbladder tract from old bile and debris, which we call stones!!"

# GASTRITIS

Digestion starts in the mouth. Have your teeth checked. Missing teeth should be replaced, so chewing can be done properly.

The lifelong request "eat slowly" has its truth. Every morsel should be mixed with saliva particularly when it is carbohydrate food.

If it is meat and meat alone you may play wolf safely because meat is prepared in the stomach, not in the mouth.

While working at Professor Brauchle's clinic he had a patient with terrible trouble in the whole digestive tract. This man had been working in Africa. It was so hot there that he only drank beer. Cold beer, he hardly ate. His intestines, including some of the stomach were all shriveled up. There Prof. Brauchle told this patient to eat meat. Not hamburger, but pieces of meat and wolf them down. No other food for 3 weeks, then a little raw vegetables could be added. Of course, no beer.

We did not believe that this man would do it. To all our astonishment he did and showed up 9 months later, a healthy man.

This gives you an illustration that meat can be gulped down

and does not have to be chewed, but all other foods should be thoroughly prepared in your mouth before swallowing.

Gastritis is an infection in the stomach. The stomach is red, inflamed, painful, and tender.

Oftentimes it goes away after a few days if you do not drink coffee, eat fat foods, fried foods, potato chips, and so on, but add Chamomile tea or a very weak tea of Ginger (spice ginger), rolled oats with a little cream or skip a meal or two.

However, there are other causes of gastritis. The stomach muscles may be weak and the whole stomach may be sagging. Not enough tone in the muscle (Hypotony). This can be helped by:

    a) improving the diet
    b) proper exercise
    c) by suggestive treatments to
       improve the will and
       joy to live.

### Chronic Gastritis

Breakfast: Oats cooked in water
eat with cream (no honey)
toast with butter (no jelly)

Midmorning: ½ glass carrot juice
½ glass milk, if possible goat's milk
mix before serving.

Lunch: Egg omelet with apple sauce
or: Egg omelet with cauliflower, soft
or: Egg omelet with broccoli, soft
or: Egg omelet with carrot, mashed
or: Baked potato with yoghurt and
vegetables and cottage cheese.

Afternoon: Herb tea with toast and butter

Evening: Yoghurt, cottage cheese, soup made from rice boiled and run through a colander, or millet done the same way.
Slowly add fish, avocado, sprouts.

In some cases patients are so weak that high protein drinks have to be given (see Health Food Stores).

After each meal:

> 3 tbsp. fresh Alfalfa juice or
> 3 tablets
> 1 cup of Rosehip tea or 250 mg.
> Rosehips

# GLANDS

### The Two-Day Diet to Stimulate Sluggish Glands

On arising: Eat ½ lb. of fruit (no bananas)

Breakfast: Have Special Soup.

### Basic Recipe for Special Soup

Boil 3 tbsp. rolled oats in 8 oz. water.
After it is done, add finely ground
parsley, caraway, sea salt, basil,
thyme or other herbs.
You may eat all you want.

Midmorning: Eat ½ lb. of fruit.

Noon: Have Special Soup. You may add stewed tomatoes, onion, leek, or fresh parsley.

Afternoon: Have two apples with almonds, nuts or roasted chestnuts.

Evening: Have either Special Soup or Bircher-Benner mush with almond milk.

Bedtime: Have ½ lb. fresh fruit if desired.

This diet is very stimulating to sluggish glands. For best results, it is done two days in a row, then repeated every ten days. See Bircher-Musli in "Recipes."

# HYPERACIDITY

One may experience belching, fullness, pressure in the stomach area and heartburn. This heartburn can come through the esophagus, even into the throat.

Heartburn is not always hyperacidity. Heartburn and fullness can happen from low acidity and also from a nervous disposition of the stomach. Don't reach all the time for the sodium bicarbonate. Change your diet so the secretions of the stomach are normalized. Good natural oils, good butter and cream and aloe vera juice are the natural stoppers of hyperacidity.

### Diet for Hyperacidity

Breakfast: Have carob drink in water with two tablespoons of heavy cream; cooked oatmeal or barley, millet or rice with butter, cream or half and half; toast with butter.

Midmorning: Eat one tablespoon ground flaxseed with a little milk or chew one tablespoon whole flaxseed slowly.

Lunch: Take mashed, boiled in-the-skin or baked potatoes; boiled, not fried, fish; cooked vegetables; salads made out of cooked vegetables. Instead of fish, you can try cottage cheese, veal, or boiled fowl or an egg dish. Do not take broth.

Midafternoon: have chamomile tear or other stomach herb tea and toast with butter.

Supper: Have cooked and mashed carrots, rice or barley or egg dish with applesauce.

Since this diet is constipating, it should be carried out no longer than ten days. Usually that is all it takes. If constipation sets in, one tablespoon of olive oil in some warm milk or juice two times a day should be added to the diet. Ground flaxseed or boilded flaxseed as a tea will also help. Food should not be too hot. Drink no ice water or any other iced food. Nothing irritates a weak stomach more than iced beverages. Soothing herb teas are calendula, chamomile, comfrey and comfrey root. Comfrey root compresses to the stomach gives a feeling of relief immediately.

# HEART AND DIET

One of the most important rules in dealing with heart-troubled patients is: Only 3 meals a day, with only fluid in between meals. No snacking. The stomach is usually enlarged and gas formation presses toward the heart. Meals should be vegetarian style, served on time. Fresh, uncooked or slightly steamed vegetables, yoghurt, cottage cheese and raw fruit are the main foods.

After 10 days some grains may be added. The stomach should rest in between meals. No fluid with meals.

In case of low heartbeat (usually after Hepatitis or when it can be traced back to that illness) following diet will restore normal heartbeat:

No food for 2 days

Make 1 gallon lime water from fresh lime to your taste. All grapesugar or honey to your taste and drink 1 cup every hour. Do this for 2 days.

## NOVEMBER 21, 1980

The ABC Network reported from a Miami convention of physicians.

These physicians emphasized that Heart Diseases are No. One Killers of America.

That the filling up of plague in the arterial system called arteriosclerosis is the underlying cause of **All Heart Diseases.**

Following formula adapted from France removes the plague in One Month.

    1 Potassium Chloride with Silica (Import)

    2 Hawthornberry Capsules

    2 Tablespoon Aloe Vera Gel in 4 ounces Fruit Juice.

Take this 3 times daily before each meal.

# JAUNDICE AND DIET

There are two kinds of jaundice. One is due to the congestion or blockage in the gall duct; and the other is due to infection. The blockage in the gall duct can be parasites or gall stones, alcohol abuse, mucous and swelling of the tissues. In any case, your physician will determine the cause. Strict diet will help. We have to direct our effort first to remove the blockage and then to get the bile washed out of the system, the blood and the tissue as fast as possible.

To remove the blockage make a cabbage or herb poultice over the liver area and give small amounts of tea, such as, Chelandonium, Chamomile, or Horsetail. Take 1-2 tablespoons every hour until the vomiting and pain stop and then give more tea. When the patient cannot keep anything down, make one cup of herb tea. Use Lobelia, or Chamomile or both. Insert the tea into the rectum. In case you have nothing in the house, pick a handful of dandelion leaves and make a tea from that.

After all the pain is gone, give your friend lots of apple juice, mixed with distilled water. Give him about a gallon a day and nothing else. The apple juice drink of ½ apple juice and ½ water, will wash the bile from the tissue, blood and glands in a hurry. It takes about 2 days.

When one has jaundice due to infection, hepatitis, buy the fruit known as limes and make yourself fresh lime water. Sweeten it with honey. This is all you get. Drink 6-8 ounces every hour, of this refreshing drink. Soon your appetite will come back and you will think of all the goodies a pastry shop has to offer. Do Not Be Tempted! Stick with the juice until you are dreadfully hungry. This might take about 2-3 days. Then break the juice diet with a small dish of cooked beets and/or cooked carrots. If you tolerate this well, you may add, 4 hours later, a piece of baked potato without butter or cream. Always drink lime water. Next day add a little fat free yoghurt or cottage cheese and some well done rice. In one week's time, you should be back on your feet.

# LYMPH

## Clean Your Lymphatic System

1 pint grapefruit juice
1 pint freshly squeezed orange juice
1 pint white grape juice
1 pint water with the juice of three limes
1 pint water with the juice of two lemons
1 pint pineapple juice
1 pint papaya juice, diluted
twelve eggs (whole)
six egg yolks
Frozen raspberries or strawberries add a
    delicious flavor.
Beat eggs and mix into fruit juice mixture.

This is one day's supply. If you are hungry, add one kind of fresh fruit.

Lymph tea consisting of:
    Red clover tops
    Chaparell
    Herb-o-lime
Available at your Health Food Store or write to author.

# MACROBIOTIC DIETS

George Osawa, the reformer and philosopher from Japan, brought to America, in the 1950's to 60's, interesting news about nutrition. Michio Kushi carries on Osawa's work. It is the philosophy of balance in food as well as in living. Concerning nutrition, the most valuable knowledge of his teaching is that male and female should be nourished a little differently. The female needs more Yin foods, such as fruits, berries and leaves. Females thrive on foods with more sugar and water content. The male thrives on salty, sour and hearty foods, such as beans and buckwheat, or Yang foods.

I go along fully with this part of the philosophy. The female should be nourished differently. Her requirements are different. For example, the female needs rice polishings, which is magnesium rich food and contains B vitamins.

The male thrives on Brewer's yeast, which is B vitamin rich food. Brewer's yeast is a highly Yang food. In addition to many B vitamins, it also carries male hormones, just as Ginseng does. Rice polishings carry female hormones, just as Dong Quai does. Dong quai is the female Ginseng. One should consider these facts by planning a diet specifically for male or female.

# LUNGS

The lung is an air organ and besides deep breathing and lots of fresh air, it needs oxygen-rich foods to stay well.

Once it becomes weakened through pneumonia, pleurisy, or other illnesses, our attention has to be fixed to all oxygen-rich foods. The best fruits are grown in the south: dates, oranges, papaya, lime, lemon, grapefruit, apricots, prickley pear, peaches. The fruit must be healthy and ripe. Other fruits do not have that much lung-healing property.

Vegetables should be raw or steamed. Sunflower oil or other good oils should be added. **Do not** cream the vegetables with flour or starch.

Green salads of wild herbs or domestic greens should be served twice. Salad dressing should be made with lemon juice, **not vinegar**, oil, spices, sea salt. If possible, serve raw vegetable juices.

People with lung congestion and weak lungs have very little appetite. Therefore, it is important that food should be served for them in a special manner.

Do not overload a plate. The patient has no courage to start. On a medium plate, pile a little cooked food in the middle and decorate the rest of the plate with greens, even nasturtium flowers or flower petals with one cherry tomato, ½ slice pickle, 1 radish cut in two.

### Schedule

Soak dried dates, apricots, figs overnight.

For Breakfast: Serve with a little cream of yoghurt.

Later On: A scrambled egg with finely cut parsley or other greens, rice cracker.

Midmorning: Raw carrot and celery juice, or fresh fruit or fruit juice.

Lunch: Baked potato, steamed vegetable with butter. Salad made with lemon juice and oil. Fish or cheese, or broiled liver, or meat, very little of it, more for decoration.

2 p.m.: 1 glass fresh fruit juice or fruit

3 p.m.: Yoghurt or buttermilk

5:30 p.m.: As at noon (but no protein)

7 p.m.: Vegetable juice or yoghurt

All lung congestion and weak lungs observe this rule: **No fluid with the meals.**

Water, herb teas between meals and/or with your vegetable and fruit juices.

In olden times lung patients were called "consumption cases" because they loose weight so easily. These people were stuffed with calorie-rich foods and ate less and less. We now know that this was wrong. Above diets not only keep the weight, but make them healthier.

Wheat products and drinking sweet milk is a No! No! in all these cases.

All lung conditions should be checked for grain allergies and milk and egg allergies. Also plants in the house can bring an allergic reaction, can constrict the nerves and there is an asthma attack.

All asthma responds at once to a teaspoon of cranberry juice concentrate. This should always be in the house available and handy, when an asthmatic is visiting your house.

The food, each one, and in combination, should be checked

for reactions. See Cook's Method or use one of the Kineisiology methods. You will be surprised to learn that some food by itself can be tolerated. However, several foods together will not be tolerated. Some foods have delayed reaction time, others react immediately.

---

**Cranberry Concentrate** to ease an asthma attack is terrific. (1 teaspoon).

---

Asthmatics should always and every day have a gallbladder tea, because the gallbladder gets easily lazy. A lazy gallbladder takes energy from lungs.

# KIDNEYS

## Diet Plan for Kidney Troubles

A great deal of attention should be placed on the kidneys. A sick kidney does not hurt, only when the sickness expands to the encasing capsules it hurts badly or when stones are passing through the kidney ducts.

A sick kidney presses upwards. It gives (a) a stiff neck, (b) disc trouble, (c) stiff and painful arms, (d) back troubles, and (e) fuzzy eyesight.

In advance cases, kidney troubles express in sore knees and finally swollen ankles.

Two-thirds of all people committed to mental institutions have kidney disorders. Some get wild, disoriented and the kidney should be checked.

The right kidney is the organ to filter inorganic substances as toxic lead, mercury, copper, D.D.T. and arsenic-bound chemicals. When overloaded, this organ does not hurt, it becomes cold to the touch (you feel it cold).

The left kidney is sensitive to infections.

### Menu
Breakfast: Chamomile and horsetail
Bircher Musli with nuts
1 slice of rye bread with butter

Midmorning: Yoghurt or buttermilk
Noon: Vegetables, raw and cooked
Salads made with oil and lemon juice, without salt
Veal, turkey, chicken, fish if boiled
Rice, millet, potatoes
Pudding if desired
Chamomile and horsetail tea.
Midafternoon: Herb tea
Fresh fruit
Evening: If hungry, as lunch, but no proteins of any kind. Better stick with fresh fruit, herb tea, bread and butter. Fruit soups are very good.

### Good Kidney Recipe

1 cup celery leaves
1 cup parsley
1½ quarts cold water

Cut celery leaves and parsley in ½ inch pieces. Put in 1½ quarts cold water. (**Not** in aluminum pot!) Simmer 20 minutes. Remove from fire, let sit for 15 minutes. Strain. Drink 8 ounces 3-4 times daily.

Twice a week take a bath in Horsetail herbs, but just sit in the water for 20 minutes, do not lay in the water, so all the blood goes into the kidney area.

Dr. Schlager (1923) recommended the following diet for several days (until the increase of urined is re-established).

Breakfast: Boil rice, or farina, or tapioca, or noodles, or cornstarch in water.
Add thick cream and serve with honey or maple sugar and applesauce or other stewed fruit.
Midmorning: Herb tea with parsley, horsetail and parsley root.
Noon: As at breakfast
Midafternoon: Herb tea
Supper: As at noon

This is a remarkable diet and has survived 60 years and has helped a lot of people suffering from kidney troubles.

After several days go to the first diet.

As your kidney recuperates slowly add chicken, veal, salads and eggs. Absolutely **forbidden** are: alcohol, nuclein-rich meats such as liver, brain, red meat, smoked meats, fish, smoked or canned, sardines, and pork. Also ready-made convenience foods are not good for the kidney.

As your physician allows it, slowly add some salt, 5 grams only (sea salt is best). Salt has to have the magnesium in it. Kelp seasons very well.

The degenerative form of kidney disease should be treated in the beginning as if the kidney is infected. Dr. Vogler's method is very, very beneficial:

Two days fasting with diluted fresh fruit juices. Apple and blueberries are best. Cherries and peach juice or cranberries in apple juice with plenty of water in it. ½ cranberry juice with ½ distilled water.

Only ½ pint of fluid should be taken at a time. After the two days, go on the nephritis diet for one week. Then slowly add cottage cheese, egg, and veal.

# NEPHRITIS AND
# THE PRIMARY AND SECONDARY
# NEPHROSCLEROSIS

The diet can not be one for all forms of kidney troubles. Let me give you some form of diet direction for the infectious type kidney problems.

### Diet for Infections in Kidneys

The main problem is that an infected kidney can not filter out the end-products of protein (end-products of protein are poisonous). The body needs protein, particularly the tissue, which becomes flabby and waterlogged and cannot handle the salt. In order to release the burden of a sick kidney (besides following your physician's prescription) **strict** diet measures are needed.

It is known that the end-products of carbohydrates and fats are carbon dioxide and water. Both can be eliminated even by a sick kidney. Therefore, our diet-form has to consist of the two, carbohydrate and water. Salt plays a terrific role in fluid retention and should be eliminated entirely for a little while.

Breakfast: Bircher-Benner Musli. It is satisfying and healing in nature. Soak 2 tbsp. rolled oats (not instant) in 6 tbsp. of water over night. To this mixture add 2 tbsp. thick cream, and 1½ apples finely grated with a little fresh lemon juice and some honey. You may substitute apples with berries, peaches, cherries, prunes, or other fruits, but do **not** use citrus fruit. As the patient gets better, the dish can be topped with 1 tbsp. finely ground nuts.

Midmorning: One orange and 1 cup herb tea as shavegrass and horsetail with 1 tsp. honey.

Lunch: Should be the heaviest meal of the day:
Rice soup or barley soup without salt
Baked potatoes, vegetable with butter and 2 egg yolks.
Pudding if desired.

Midafternoon: Herb tea as midmorning
Fresh fruits: pears and apples

Supper: Yoghurt, buttermilk, vegetables, rice. Everything without salt. Season with herbs, parsley, thyme, chives, tarragon, sage, green onion.

Bedtime: Fresh fruit juice with water.

### Fasting for Kidney Ailments

Boil crushed watermelon seeds—1 cup to 3 quarts water for 3 minutes. Strain and store 2 quarts in refrigerator, while leaving the rest on the table. Every hour take ⅓ cup of this luke warm tea. For breakfast take watermelon, for lunch acidophilus milk, and/or yoghurt, vegetable and raw food, some fish or egg, and rye bread. Supper is stewed pears or applesauce with yoghurt or soy milk, as much as you like. Do this diet for three days but continue watermelon seed tea and watermelon breakfasts for fourteen days.

This recipe comes from Turkey. It was given to my mother by a prominent religious authority. I have given away this recipe many times. Every time the result was immediate and astounding. It balances the fluids in the system by releasing electrical currents and re-establishing the yin-yang function of the kidney.

**Kidney:** smartweed tea or beet, ½ tsp., and 1 heaping tsp. parsley to 1 cup water.

70

# NERVES

## Three Days for Better Nerves

It takes willpower and authority to stay on a diet, especially when your nerves give out.

Following routine only three days in a row will make a better "boss," a stronger personality out of you. After that, one day a week or one day every two weeks will keep your nerves sweet.

In one pint of cottage cheese, mix three tablespoons almond oil or safflower oil and two egg yolks. Mix well and either make it sweet with honey, or spicy with onions, salt and herbs. Also boil four tablespoons of barley in two quarts of water for 35 minutes. Strain and add honey and lime or lemon juice to the barley water so it tastes good.

Before Breakfast: 1 cup of warm barley water
    Breakfast: Prepared cottage cheese and carrots, raw or cooked.
    Midmorning: Barley water
    Noon: Steamed zucchini, cooked green beans, and cottage cheese, spices
    Midafternoon: Barley water
    Evening: Cottage cheese, zucchini stewed or baked in the oven. Dish of barley. Carrot salad. Barley water.
    Bedtime: Barley water and calcium tablets.

# MUCOUS CLEANSER

A diet to clear mucous out of intestines. This was donated to this book by a chiropractor in Los Angeles.

It is amazing to see the amount of mucous leaving the body, in people you never suspected had this trouble.

> Buy unfiltered apple juice, for bulk use
>> psyllium seeds
>> or mucovada
>> or Intesto-Klenz
>> or ground flax seeds
>
> Buy also: papaya tablets
>> pancreatin
>> fenugreek (to have on hand.)

## Schedule

7:00 a.m.  1 glass distilled water with 1 tsp. bulk
(mentioned above)

1 glass Apple juice with 1 papaya tablet

1 pancreatin

1 comfrey and pepsin

1 cup fenugreek tea

Continue to do this by the following schedule: Take the above at 7:00 a.m., 9:00 a.m. 11:00 a.m., 1:00 p.m., 3:00 p.m., 5:00 p.m. and at 8:00 p.m.

Every time you drink the apple juice, take pancreatin and so on. Take an herbal laxative if needed or an enema with chamomile tea. This diet should be kept up for 3-4 days. It will also release sinus conditions, since it loosens all the mucous in the body.

# MUCOUS CLEANSER

for: Sinus
for: Stomach
for: Lungs
for: Bronchii

For two days drink nothing but freshly squeezed oranges followed by the same amount of distilled water.

Drink slowly 6-8 ounces fresh Orange Juice followed by 6-8 ounces distilled water.

One or 2 hours later do the same thing. The more you drink the better it is. You can have it as often as 15 times a day but not less than 5 times a day.

Do not mix juice and water. It has to be taken as indicated. I have seen sinus condition dry up like magic. Cough disappear, headache vanish, and so on.

# PANCREAS

## Diet Plan for the Pancreas

A diet plan for a malfunctioning pancreas depends on the findings of your physician. What specifically is wrong? Is it:

a. Impairment due to faulty enzyme functions of the pancreas.

b. Trouble with the Island of Langerhans. (Diabetes)

Let us talk about the first part. The pancreas sends digestive juices, or digestive enzymes, into the intestines. These enzymes are needed for fat digestion and protein digestion. Some people have lots of flatuence, or gas. No matter what they eat, the abdomen swells. Sometimes they may even find fat gobules swimming in the toilet bowl. This shows that these poor people suffer a lot. Their fat intake should then consist of emulsified fats, as in egg yolk, oil emulsified in a blender with lemon juice and water or yoghurt, or cream emulsified in juice or water. All fats have to be at low, low levels until the glands recuperate.

In case the protein digestion enzyme is the trouble maker, then all proteins have to be taken in predigestive form and papaya enzyme given.

Usually both the protein and fat digestion enzymes are im-

74

paired. Therefore the diet becomes a problem. In such case, give "Strawberry and Banana Diet" for one or two days; then every ten days. This is a real help. It is amazing how well this combination is tolerated.

## Liver-Pancreas Stimulant

Take ½ teaspoon nutmeg in 1 cup hot water. This causes the pancreas to release juices and will rebuild the liver.

## Pep Drink

Blend sunflower seeds, dates and water.

## Schedule

Several small meals have to be offered. Care hs to be taken that only fat-free cheeses, chicken (no skin), and skim milk (no whole milk) are given.

Breakfast: Have rolled oats boiled in water served with one teaspoon of honey, one glass of skim milk, and one slice of toast with jelly. Anise toast is well tolerated.

Midmorning: Have stewed or raw fruit, whatever is best tolerated.

Lunch: Boil beef in plenty of water. Remove all fat from the broth and also the meat. Now boil rice or barley in the broth. When it is done, take the pan from the fire and finely cut parsley, some sprouts, and caraway into the soup. Vegetable, potatoes, and some fish. Chicken or turkey meat is allowed.

Midafternoon: Skim milk or herb tea, with toast and jelly should be taken.

Early
Evening Meal: Have vegetable soup and one hour later, fat-free yoghurt. If still hungry at bedtime, have skim milk and toast and jelly.

Every 10 days the patient should have strawberries and bananas, eaten together, all they want to eat for one day. It is amazing how well it is tolerated.

IMPORTANT: Do Not Drink Liquid With Your Meals!

A normal functioning of the enzyme production of the pancreas is largely dependent upon proper hydrochloric acid secretion of the stomach. Fluids during meals dilute this acid. Conversely, with the help of small amounts of hydrochloric acid after meals, the pancreatic action is increased and normalized. Comfrey and pepsin is a natural.

Green beans seasoned with sage, sea salt, and parsley is a specific in a sick pancreas. Also drink the water the green beans were cooked in.

In case the insulin secretion of the pancreas is also in trouble, more fat-free protein has to be given, and enough insulin to get this under control. See physician.

Insufficient secretion of the pancreas brings gas and discomfort. Pancreatin tablets can be bought at Healthfood Stores to relieve this.

# PREGNANCY AND DIET

Dr. V. Noorden estimated the needed calorie intake of pregnancy between 2nd and 5th month to be 150 calories and later on 300-400 calories, over the need of the mother. That is not very much, however the quality of food is important.

While speaking of quality we think of proteins, but in pregnancy this is not the way to go. The unborn needs minerals as calcium, iron magnesium, zinc and the whole row of traceminerals, organic and inorganic. For instance it was calculated that the fetus needs 34 grams of pure calcium to develop properly.

If there is not enough calcium the new, developing body will rob it from the mother.

When in pregnancy a mother refrains from salt, she can drink all the fluids she wants without causing edema.

The following recipe has helped many from pregnancy-intoxications.

1 level teaspoon Epsom salt in 6 ounces water every hour, 4 times. That will relieve the danger at once. Whenever albumin shows in the urine, the mother should not drink milk. Diluted fruit juices, water and vegetable juices are to be taken.

The normal development of the child is dependent on the presence of enought viatmins as: A, B-comples, C-complex, E₊and D.

Vitamin E, 100 units for the baby is a must.

Vitamin A best through carrots.

Therefore, in the state of pregnancy, every woman should have vitamins and mineral supplemets and good natural foods, vegetable, fruit, whole grain and supplements.

# MORNING SICKNESS

Take 1 cup Peach Tree Leaf Tea with 50 Mg. B-6, twice daily (1 tsp. to 1 cup hot water), also, increase Zinc intake.

Breakfast: a. 2 eggs with salad
b. oats cooked in water with fresh fruit
c. raw oats with fruit and skim milk
peppermint-chamomile tea

Midmorning: An apple or a tomato

Lunch: If possible have a late lunch. Have fish or lean meat with salad and vegetables. Have oil and vinegar dressing. No mayonnaise.

Midafternoon: Apples and oranges

Evenings: Cottage cheese
Salad, vegetables
Yoghurt, kefir
Rice, millet

Especially recommended at herb teas are:

Lady's Mantle, it relieves the overactive pancreas and curbs the appetite. Peppermint-chamomile gives a feeling of satisfaction. Hawthorn tea is good for circulation. Season your food with kelp and dulse. They are thyroid food. Sprinkle plenty of fresh parsley on your vegetables to increase your kidney action. If needed, a cup of kidney tea does wonders. Sprinkle cayenne pepper over your food for better circulation. Mix paprika with your cottage cheese to give pep to all your sluggish glands. Be sure to take a vitamin-mineral supplement. Cayenne, kelp and hawthorn are also in tablet form in case you don't like the taste.

# PHLEBITIS AND DIET

Eat sparingly.
Drink plenty of diluted fruit juices, 6 oz. juice to 2 oz. water.
Buy unfiltered apple juice, for bulk use
    psyllium seeds
    or mucovada
    or Intesto-Klenz
    or ground flax seeds
Buy also: papaya tablets
        pancreatin
        fenugreek (to have on hand.)

## Schedule

7:00 a.m.   1 glass distilled water with 1 tsp. bulk
                      (mentioned above)
           1 glass Apple juice with 1 papaya tablet
           1 pancreatin
           1 comfrey and pepsin
           1 cup fenugreek tea

Continue to do this by the following schedule: Take the above at 7:00 a.m., 9:00 a.m., 11:00 a.m., 1:00 p.m., 3:00 p.m., 5:00 p.m. and at 8:00 p.m.

Every time you drink the apple juice, take pancreatin and so on. Take an herbal laxative if needed or an enema with chamomile tea. This diet should be kept up for 3-4 days. It will also release sinus conditions, since it loosens all the mucous in the body.

# STOMACH

The following foods are particularly healing to sick stomachs, to ulcers, pain, discomfort and sufferings from stomach distress.

| | |
|---|---|
| carrot | okra |
| coconut milk | egg white |
| egg plant | parsnip |
| flaxseed tea | sweet potato |
| slippery elm tea with cream | cottage cheese |
| goats milk | aloe vera juice, best of all |

Take no grapefruit in stomach trouble.

## Ulcer Diet

If you are in a hurry to be healed from stomach ulcers, follow the carrot diet:

Boil a good portion of carrots in pure water, without aluminum of any kind, neither pots, pans, nor foil.

When the carrots are done you eat them in different styles:

Take a napkin and eat them rabbit style,

Mash them to puree, or

Broil them after they are cooked, or

Make a soup pureed, or

Slice them lengthwise or square.

No butter, no salt. That is all you eat for 7 days. Twice a day you may have 6 ounces raw carrot juice, either with 2 tablespoons cream or with 6 ounces goatmilk.

In Europe there are special resorts for healing stomach ulcers, and this is their diet:

For the first days nothing but carrots, cooked and mashed.

On the fourth day—

Morning: carrot soup
Midmorning: potato broth
Noon: potato and carrot
Midafternoon: herb tea & cream and rice crackers
Evening: carrots and baked potato
Bedtime: herb tea & cream

One week on this regime and most of the people can increase their food intake to a normal protective diet.

Avoid all aluminum, in pots, pans or foil, the electromagnetic field is disturbed.

# REVITALIZING DIET

After eating a lifetime of wrong food combinations, poisoned by chemicals, additives and no energy, your body rebels. Nothing works any longer. The eyes give out. Everything hurts. The blood pressure plays escalator (up and down with every mood). The heart pounds and shortness of breath begins. In short, you are going to pieces! Now is the time to think of doing something fundamental, something that will change your life. something that turns the ship around!

Saturday morning make your decision for one week and two days, and these will be the best nine days of your life.

7 a.m.    4 ounces sauerkraut juice
          4 ounces tomatoe juice
8 a.m.    6-7 ounces hot lemon juice
9 a.m.    6-7 ounces hot vegetable broth
10 a.m.* 6-7 ounces cool grapefruit juice

Change every hour. Hot and cold, broth hot, grapefruit cool.

# SENIOR DIABETES

The slowing down processes of the Pancreas is the true factor of aging. As we increase the number of birthdays, the insulin-pancreatic juices diminish in quantity and quality because the pancreas shrinks. Particularly if you accumulated aluminum-lead in your system this pancreas shrinking process goes very very fast. You age before your time.

First goes the eyesight, you have to have glasses because "sugar crystals" settle in eyes. You cannot recall your memories, names and so on. Your thinking slows down. You start having pains in legs, discoloration of legs and feet. You showel your walk and sleep is disturbed.

All this shows that your trouble is real even so a urine or blood test will not indicate Diabetis.

No sugar, cakes, cookies, no shortcut in food preparation, no T.V. dinners.

Lots of Vegetables, 5 different kinds a day. Protein for breakfast and lunch.

No protein at night. And consider taking D-Bets, which is total food for the pancreas (ask author)

Tryptophane, Zinc, Chromium and Multi Mineral and Vitamins.

In all forms of Senior diabetes, the liver function should be supported also. The liver carries an extra burden when the pancreas gets weak. The whole group of B vitamins with extra choline and inositol should be incorporated in the diet plan.

# TUMOR DIET TO BRING
# OXYGEN TO TISSUES

Breakfast: Bircher-Musli with cottage cheese and oil.

Midmorning: Seeds

Lunch: Eggplant and kelp and cottage cheese. Take an eggplant and peel very thick. Do not use the inside of the eggplant. Boil or bake it. Mash it thoroughly and add kelp and **freshly ground** pepper. Kelp is important, but if you dislike kelp on the food, take 4 kelp tablets with the meal.

You can also bake the whole eggplant. When done, discard the inside and mash the rest thoroughly.

Take 1 pint cottage cheese and blend it with finely cut onions, parsley or rosemary, or sage, sea salt and 2 tbsp. sunflower seed oil.

Supper: Beet soup or a beet dish

Onion soup: Red and white onions are cut in small pieces. Saute them on low heat with a little butter. Add coarse-cut potato peelings and celery. If you have string bean

water left over, take that or add water
seasoned with sea salt.

## Second Day
Breakfast: Bircher-Musli with cottage cheese.
   Noon: Green beans cooked with potato peelings
(coarsely-peeled potatoes)
Cottage cheese with seeds, beet salad
   Supper: Baked eggplant: Peel eggplants 1 inch
around. Soak them in salt water to take out
the bitterness, for about 1 hour.
Then place them in an oiled baking dish with
red and white onions and slices of tomatoes.
Season with kelp or sea salt. If no kelp is
used, 4 kelp tablets with each meal.
Salad

## Fourth Day
Breakfast: Granola with cream and water
Cottage cheese sweetened with honey and
1 slice of dark bread or cottage cheese with
herbs piled high on the dark bread.
   Lunch: Eggplant caviar, onion soup (as above)
Salad, 1 slice rye bread or cornbread
Cottage cheese sweetened or salty
   Supper: Baked red and white onions
Cornmeal mush (Polenta), with stewed to-
matoes and salad dish

## Fifth Day
Breakfast: Cornmeal mush or musli
Cottage cheese preparation
   Lunch: Rye bread with cottage cheese
preparation
Onion soup as above
Salad

Supper: Again baked eggplant peels with red nd
white onions
Cornbread
Salad

### Sixth and Seventh Days
Breakfast: Cornmeal mush or musli with cottage cheese
mixed with honey or herbs.
Lunch: From the dishes given. If you serve musli
in the morning, give cornbread for lunch.
Millet allowed and very good.
Seeds with meal or in-between meals.
Always cottage cheese mixture for lunch and
salad twice a day.

# DR. CUHL'S CANCER DIET

This researcher is very well known and his findings are well founded. The result is excellent.

He improves cell respiration by giving cold pressed oils in salads, cottage cheese and in vegetables. He gives yoghurt, sauerkraut, cottage cheese and kefir, buttermilk, fermented vegetable juices, and in particular, fermented beet juice. Vegetables and fruits should be organically grown, i.e., without spray or artificial fertilizers. Carbohydrates, sugar and potatoes are not on the menu. Some eggs and fowl are permitted.

### Enzyme Diet

| | |
|---|---|
| When you first get out of bed in the morning: | Drink diluted cherry juice or lemon juice and water or cranberry with lemon peel, soaked overnight. |
| Breakfast: | Have hormone breakfast with fruit |
| or: | flax seed ground up |
| or: | barley with honey, cream and fruit |
| or: | millet cereal with cream and cottage cheese with oil |
| or: | a slice of whole wheat bread. |

Lunch: Have cooked vegetables and a raw vegetable salad

or: cottage cheese seasoned and enriched with oil, such as sunflower oil

or: fish or chicken or lamb

Afternoon: Fruit and whole wheat toast if wanted.

Supper: Have raw salad, rice or baked potato and yoghurt

Have this each day for supper. You may also have eggplant with kelp.

# HOW TO FEED
# A PERSON WITH TUMORS

First consideration: Diet should be changed every week.

1. 7 days a diet to clean out the intestine from accumulated waste, including parasites. (See Clay Diet)
2. Diet to remove environmental toxins—3 days only. (See Environmental Toxin Diet)
3. Diet to reduce the size of tumor and bring oxygen into the tissues. (See Oxygen Diet)
4. Diet to bring as many enzymes to the body as possible. (See Enzyme Diet)
5. Diet to maintain health. (See Energy Diet)

### Eggplant with Kelp

Take an eggplant and peel it so that it is very thick. Boil the thick peelings and when they are done, mash them until pulp-like. Add kelp to this pulp. Eat ½ cup once or twice a day, every day. Its healing properties are remarkable.

Be sure you also eat some asparagus every day. Several tablespoonsful will do. Do not eat protein after 2 p.m.

After the Tumor is gone one has to rebuild the resistance of tissue, muscles, glands, organs so a tumor can **never** return.

America has one type of grape which has the **rebuilding healing** power in it. It is the Concord grape.

Take 36 ounces of Concord grape juice

Add 4 ounces distilled water

Drink this in following fashion for 6 weeks:

In small sips from 8 a.m.-11 a.m.

No tea, water, coffee, no food allowed.

Between 11 a.m.-12 noon **nothing** to drink or eat. 12 noon a good lunch with plenty of protein, vegetables, salads. For supper take carbohydrates as rice, bread, potatoes, millet, corn with vegetables and salads. Fruits between lunch and supper.

# REDUCING DIETS

## Overeating

Most weight problems are caused by eating too much of things we don't need and often not enough of what we do need. Often, our urges to eat (and overeat) come from:

1. mineral deficiencies
2. enzyme deficiencies
3. parasites
4. emotional problems
5. glandular disturbances
6. over-tiredness

Our overeating urges almost always come from two or more of above mentioned causes.

# OVERWEIGHT

50 years ago the famous "Karell" treatment for overweight conditions was done in hospitals. It consists of taking, in the morning, 8 ounces of milk, 5 times and 1 teaspoon of epsom salts in 1 glass of water. At night, take fruit. Enemas were given 2 times a day and the patient was supervised in the hospital. This was done for 4-6 days.

This treatment of freeing the body of trapped sodium, water and wastes is too harsh for a working person. However, for one day a week, lets say Sunday, it is safe and sound, provided you get lots of rest.

Another version of the Karell treatment, also done in hospitals, was ½ pound of fruit, 5 times a day. This was also done with enemas, rest and laxative teas if needed. This is much easier to take and instead of one week in the hospital, Saturday and Sunday at home, with lots of rest, does wonders.

After the initial cleanup day of either fruit or milk, a low calorie diet should follow. Never plan a reducing diet for only one week or one month. The endocrine system is at low gear and the glands have to be nourished and re-established to full capacity. That takes time. Plan to loose 5 pounds a month, initially more. That makes 60 pounds in a year. This is a safe and sound diet plan for the heart and all the organs, also for your pocket book, for you'll need new clothes.

The reason for a crash diet, initially, for one or two days is that the ballooned stomach has a chance to shrink, thus the hunger feeling of a low calorie diet will be lessened.

Here are several reducing diets.

# DIETS

When we think of diets, we always think first of reducing diets. There are "crash diets" which often come and go with the seasons. Here are some classics, which you may already know and might like to try:

### The Milk and Banana Diet
Eat four bananas and drink three 8 ounce glasses of skim milk each day. It's best to start the day with a banana and then alternate skim milk and banana throughout the day.

### The Yoghurt Diet
Eat four cups of plain yoghurt and one medium cantaloupe each day.

### The Apple-A-Meal Diet
For those more concerned with a diet's ease than speed. Dr. Neil Solomon, a weight-control specialist, recommends that you eat whatever you want, but cut the portions in half; and before each meal drink an 8 ounce glass of water and eat an apple. Dr. Solomon believes that the apple and water combination introduces calories to the body that signal the brain to

turn off its appetite alarm. They also help the dieter feel full, so eating half-portions is easier. Assuming the individual is eating nutritiously, Dr. Solomon says his apple-a-meal regimen is safe and effective for losing an average of five pounds per month.

### The Soup Diet

For lunch **slowly** spoon a bowl of soup. Afterwards eat a salad chewing thoroughly. Do this four or five times a week. The results are slow but sure and there are no harmful effects.

### Reducing Diet with Potatoes

The potato has 20% carbohydrate and an appreciable amount of trace minerals, particularly calcium and a good supply of vitamin C.

In contrast to all other tuber vegetables, the potato has a complete protein. It is very little, only 1.5% but this protein, has all 8 essential amino acids. The nutritional value of a potato depends a great deal on the soil the tuber is grown in. When the soil is rich in minerals, the potato will pick up an abundance of minerals. The potato feels heavy in the hand and the grocery sack is only half full, however, you are buying a tasty and mineral and protein rich product.

If a potato is grown on an artificially over-supplied, fertilized soil, the potato will be huge and juicy if enough fluid was supplied, but the taste is not exquisite as a homegrown potato.

Potatoes remain in the stomach for 2½ hours, rice only one hour. The satisfying value in a potato is to be appreciated, also. Potatoes are easily digestible, if they are mashed with a fork or thoroughly chewed. potatoes have a non-irritating bulk and are therefore excellent in bowel trouble and good for a sensitive and an irritated digestive tract.

Potatoes have an insulin-like hormone, which helps to digest the 20% carbohydrates it has.

Contrary to all beliefs, the potato is not fattening. It is the gravy, the sour cream, the butter which goes with the potato that makes it a no-no food in dieting.

If you decide to lose weight, try a potato diet. Find good potatoes in your grocery store. Hold them in your hand to weigh and compare the different kinds. The heavier they feel, the better they are. Avoid potatoes where skin is turning green.

Do not peel them. By peeling and boiling them as we all used to do it, we throw 75% of the minerals down the drain.

Potatoes should be steamed or baked in the oven, do not use aluminum foil. The wrapping of aluminum foil hinders the body to utilize the protein and minerals of the potato and since you have nothing but the potatoes to eat, this becomes important.

## Rice Diet for Water-Logged Condition

Take one cup brown rice. (Short grain is to be preferred, because it has more minerals.) Wash it and put it in two cups boiling water, without salt. Boil for thirty-five minutes on low heat. This kind of rice is to be eaten whenever one is hungry. At noon and night, some applesauce or stewed pears, without sugar, might be added. Or you may boil some wheat germ and middlings in water and use as you would the above recipe. For best results use it five to seven days.

How and why does this diet work? When the sodium, which is in the fluid surrounding the cell, comes in disharmony with the potassium, which is supposed to be in the cell, fluid builds up. The fluid is kept in proper proportion and harmony through the positive and negative electricity of the two opponents and components, sodium and potassium. When the sodium decides to pay a visit to the potassium in the cell, the potassium will leave. The sodium, which has no business in the cell, cannot handle the incoming fluid, and you start to be water-logged.

## Special Help for Glands While Dieting
### Adrenal Glands

Our adrenal glands are natural weight controllers. Every food that nourishes the adrenal glands acts as a weight reducer.

## Sample Light Diet
### 800-1000 Calories

Breakfast: 1 oz. of bran and wheat germ with skim milk or a small dish of oatmeal or two eggs with a salad.
1 slice of dry whole wheat toast
1 piece of fresh fruit
1 cup of herb tea if desired

Midmorning: 1 orange or apple

Lunch: 1 medium salad with 1 tbsp. of oil mixed into the dressing or a medium raw vegetable dish.
1 medium square of corn bread or rye crisps or melba toast
1 cup of vegetable broth
6 oz. of vegetable juice
1 cup of herb tea if desired

Midafternoon: fruit

Supper: 1 medium salad with at least four fresh vegetables with 1 tbsp. of oil mixed into the dressing.
1 bowl of light soup or 1 bowl of steamed vegetables
1 small portion of cottage cheese
4 oz. vegetable juice
1 cup herb tea if desired

# A SAMPLE 7-DAY MENU PLAN

## Monday

Breakfast: ½ grapefruit
2 eggs, boiled or poaches
1 apple, slice or grated
tea or coffee
skim milk, 4 ounces in peppermint tea is
very refreshing and satisfying

Lunch: Tuna fish, 3-4 ounces
with a nice salad of mixed vegetables such
as cucumber, tomato, lettuce and more.
Have a dill-vinegar dressing over the salad

Midafternoon: 4 ounces yoghurt

Dinner: Chicken, 4-5 ounces
Salad and vegetables
Brown rice or ½ potato

## Tuesday

Breakfast: Bircher-Musli with fresh fruit, if possible,
in season.
4 ounces skim milk
1 slice whole wheat bread with 1 tsp. butter
Tea

Lunch: 2 slices rye bread
2 ounces cheese
Salad of sprouts, lettuce, tomatoes and spinach with oil-vinegar dressing
Snack: A pear or an orange
Dinner: 8 fl. oz. mixed vegetable juice
4-6 oz. broiled fish
10 spears asparagus
4 oz. baked butternut squash
1 tsp. margarine
Green salad
1 tsp. vegetable oil
4 fl. oz. skim milk
Beverage

### Wednesday

Breakfast: Orange juice
Cottage cheese with fresh fruit
Peppermint tea with or without milk
Lunch: 2 hard boiled eggs, or 4 oz. salmon or other fish
Tomato wedges and cucumber slices
Cole slaw
Beverage
Baked or raw apple if desired
Snack: Hot carob drink with a slice of whole wheat bread or 2 graham crackers.
Supper: 4-6 oz. broiled veal
½ cup brown rice
1 tsp. margarine
½ cup zucchini
Romaine salad
1 tsp. vegetable oil
½ cup apple sauce
4 fl. oz. skim milk
Beverage

## Thursday

Breakfast: 1 large piece of melon with peanut butter
Rolled oats cereal with skim milk and honey

Lunch: 8 fl. oz. tomato juice
3-4 oz. sardines
1 slice pumpernickle bread
pickle, celery and carrot strips
apple or apple sauce
4 fl. oz. skim milk
beverage

Snack: 6 fl. oz. buttermilk

Dinner: 4-6 oz. broiled liver
4 oz. onions
½ cup cauliflower
lettuce wedge
2 tsp. vegetable oil
beverage

## Friday

Breakfast: Bircher-Musli with 4 oz. skim milk
1 slice whole wheat bread with 1 tsp. butter
beverage

Lunch: mushroom omelet (2 eggs)
green salad
1 tsp. vegetable oil
baked apple or applesauce
5 oz. humburger

Dinner: ½ cup broccoli
½ cup corn
1 tsp. margarine
endive salad
1 tsp. vegetable oil
beverage

## Saturday

Breakfast: ½ cup blueberries or other berries
1 oz. uncooked cereal

4 fl. oz. skim milk
beverage

Lunch: vegetable soup with 1 frankfurter
1 slice apple pie or yoghurt

Dinner: 4-6 oz. shrimp
4 oz. Brussel sprouts
1 tsp. margarine
½ cup eggplant
tossed salad
1 tsp. vegetable oil
8 fl. oz. skim milk
beverage

### Sunday

Breakfast: Pick one of the breakfast menus you liked best.

Lunch: 3-4 oz. roast turkey
4 oz. baked acorn swuash
½ cup string beans
2 tsp. margarine
beverage

Snack: ½ cup fresh fruit salad

Dinner: 4-6 oz. broiled steak
sliced tomatoes on lettuce
1 tsp. mayonnaise
vegetables
½ medium cantaloupe
beverage
Youth: add 8 fl. oz. skim milk
Men: 6-8 oz. broiled steak

### Overweight Drink

2 tsp. Tamari sauce
½ tsp. kelp
2 tsp. lecithin
1 cup water

Make several cups and place in a bottle. Drink as you desire, all day long.

# SPECIFIC HEALING PROPERTIES
# IN FOODS

**Apples:** Whatever ails you; gallbladder trouble, liver trouble, diarrhea, tooth decay, constipation, loss of appetitie; good as poultice, too. When someone is very ill, take an apple and scrape the meat with a silver spoon. You will see them recover.

**Apricots:** Detoxify the liver and pancreas.

**Asparagus:** For fatty tumors and the like. Helpful in urinary secretions.

**Anise:** For flatulent conditions.

**Avocado:** A fat and protein supplier. Good for the diabetic.

**Barley:** A calcium supplier, colon aid and lymph cleanser.

**Aduki Beans:** For kidney trouble and swelling of ankles.

**Beans and Corn:** Muscle builders.

**Green Beans:** Removes metallic poison. Good for the malfunctions of the pancreas.

**Lima Beans:** Make a dish with lima beans, bell peppers and sweet potato to combat drug residue.

**Red Beans:** A muscle builder. Served with corn, it is a complete protein.

**White Beans:** For the eyes and liver trouble.

**Black Bean Juice:** For hoarseness and laryngitis.

**Blackberries:** Colon food. For diarrhea.

**Blueberries:** Feed the pancreas, for sugar problems.

**Blueberry and Banana:** Pancreatitis.

**Buckwheat:** For energy and warmth. For strong muscles.

**Cranberry:** A kidney food. Releases sudden cramps as in asthma and the like.

**Strawberries:** A skin berry, cleanser.

**Strawberry and Squash:** Removes metallic poisons, arsenic.

**Cherries:** For gout.

**Cherries (Sour):** For gout and as a blood cleanser.

**Grapes:** Anti-tumor, good for anemia and aura builder.

**Beef:** Muscle food.

**Beets:** Spleen food.

**Bell Pepper:** Eyes and Digestion (increases pepsin).

**Butternut:** Liver food.

**Cabbage:** For Viamin U, the tissue builder.

**Carrots:** Eyes, blood and lymph.

**Celery:** A low-calorie reducing aid.

**Celery Seed:** Drink the tea for obesity.

**Chicken:** A gland food.

**Chickpeas:** A gland food. Good protein. An anti-virus, particularly anti-polio virus.

**Crab Apple:** For vertigo.

**Cucumber:** As skin remedy, kidney cleanser; an infection cleanser.

**Currants:** Build resistance to colds. For anemia.

**Eggplant:** Give to the afflicted tumor, the peelings and dulse.

**Figs:** A de-wormer.

**Fish:** Good protein and iodine supplier.

**Garlic:** Carbohydrate residue in tissue and glands.

**Grapefruit:** A lime supplier. A flu destroyer.

**Indian Corn:** Perfect food for man. Has all the energies, amino acids and hormones the body needs.

**Kale:** Gives resistance to colds.

**Leek:** For reducing. A pancreas food, tissue builder and brain food.

**Lemon:** Vitamin C.

**Lemon (The White):** Bioflavenoid. Strengthens tissue.

**Lentils:** Iron. Contains protein supplies of the best quality.

**Lime:** For yellow jaundice.

**Meat:** Lots of calories. Protein that gives an explosive energy. Appetite satisfying.

**Millet:** Meat of the vegetarian. 15% protein.

**Black Strap Molasses:** A mineral and iron supplier.

**Oats:** Brain food.

**Oils, Cold Pressed:** Needed to assimilate the proteins from vegetables. Also a kidney food.

**Okra:** Regulates female bleeding. Gives strength to leukemic patients.

**Okra and Apples:** For ulceration of the stomach.

**Onions:** Make a soup of fresh red and white onions and collards for the flu.

**Oranges:** Has vitamin C for flu prevention.

**Papaya:** For protein digestion.

**Parsnip:** For intolerance to milk.

**Parsley:** For piles.

**Parsley Root:** For kidneys. When boiled in white wine it is for the heart.

**Peaches:** Good during pregnancy.

**Pears:** Kidney and colon.

**Peas:** Green and dried peas are a good source of protein and good for weak stomachs.

**Pineapple:** Enzyme supplier.

**Pomegranate:** A de-wormer.

**Red Potatoes:** For stomach and duodenal ulcer.

**Potato Peelings:** For kidney ailments.

**Prunes:** Iron, constipation.

**Pumpkin:** De-wormer. Parasite, spleen and pancreas food.

**Radishes:** In small amounts, promotes bile flow.

**Raisins:** Anemia, blood builder.

**Rhubarb:** Colon cleanser.

**Rice:** Universal acceptance by all tissue (over-rated at the present time).

**Rice Gruel:** Diarrhea.

**Romaine Lettuce:** Virus infection.

**Rutabaga:** Food for prayer. Feeds friendly bacteria in colon. once a week it would be good.

**Rye:** Muscle builder.

**Sesame Seeds:** Complete amino acid supplier. Makes strong-willed people. Supplies osmium, a trace mineral.

**Sauerkraut:** Keeps old folk's ailments away.

**Spinach:** Good for you if you have anemia.

**Sunflower Seeds:** Feeds eyes, sinuses and glands.

**Sweet Potato:** Gland food.

**Swiss Chard:** Arthritis (Contains Wulzen factor).

**Tomato:** As poultices in deep-rooted afflictions. When stewed, good for liver. Fresh tomatoes are a Vitamin C supplier. Green tomatoes in very small quantities are a gland stimulant. Always remove the core and stem. Make a deep insertion. This stem part is poisonous.

**Turnips:** For deep-rooted tumors. For deep-rooted resentments.

**Watercress:** Vitamin C and E supplier.

**Watermelon:** For sluggish kidney and a kidney cleanser.

**Wheat:** Starch and calorie supplier.

**Yams:** Hormone food.

**Yoghurt:** Intestinal health.

# GEMS

Arthritis............Oil of wintergreen to joints, also kerosene to joints. Eat strawberries, cranberries and asparagus.

Athletes foot.......Red beet, spinach seed, celery seed and celery.

Brain food.........Osmium (trace mineral), squash, raspberries, sesame seeds, Indian corn.

Cancer of tongue .Galium verum 3, Ladies bed straw, symphytum officinales (comfrey root)

Fallout .............Causticum (homeopathic remedy)

Cataract............Lithium dissolves cataract, natural cheddar cheese.

Clots................Cerebral embolism solvents are: Vitamin F, lecithin, cactus syrup and liquid chlorophyll

Colds ...............Fresh onions, red and white.

Drug residue ......Green sweet bell pepper, sweet potato peel, green pepper whole and lima bean pods.

Fungus.............Speia and Bryonia-Gelsemium (homeopathic remedies). Fungus grows in alkaline medium; natural antibiotics are: grapefruit, garlic, willow, parsley and radish, chlorophyll and bee pollen.

Gangrene...........Raw mashed tomatoes every two hours over the feet (or over the gangrene). 1 hour rest. Leave on all night.
Poultice of tobacco leaves, crushed. Heals in 10 days.

Infection............Garlic drink: cut cloves of garlic fine and pour hot milk over it, let stand for 10 minutes and serve before you go to bed.

Gout.................Apples for gout.
Deep massage in small of back.

Involuntary Nervous
System...........Ginseng works on it.

Hernia...............Mistletoe and horsetail.

Inflamation of
the Colon........Irish potato peel
Flax seed meal

Intestinal
Disorder.........1 cup aloe vera, 1 quart water
juice of 1 grapefruit, 3 oranges, 1 lemon
3 tbsp. milksugar, honey to taste
or: Honey to taste. 1 grapefruit, 1 lemon
3 tbsp. milk sugar, 1 quart water
½ cup aloe vera juice

Itchy Skin..........Marjoram

High Blood
Pressure.........Carbomide and lemon and orange juice

Malaria..............Collard seed, parsley seed, red pepper seed

⅓ of all Nervous Diseases have Kidney Trouble — Use horse tail.

Parasitic virus,
Microscopic
organism.........Lima bean pods, peach tree leaves

The **Parotid Gland** is connected with leukemia, and is involved in cystic fibrosis, uterine fibroids and ovarian cysts.

Pneumonia.........Parsley and seeds
Protein putrefacation end product
Spinach seed, spinach and garlic
Carbohydrate end product
Lemon juice and peel and garlic
Collard seed, carrot tops, leeks and epsom salts baths

Intestinal
Difficulties ......Potato drink: Boil 2 medium potatoes, cut in pieces in 1 quart water, with peeling; pour 4 cups of potato water over 3 tbsp. flax seed (ground) and 6 tbsp. bran. Let stand overnight and serve it warm for breakfast with lemon or orange juice and a small, finely chopped onion, it tastes good and is more nutritious.

Ulceration of
Intestines........Potatoes, garlic and golden seal

Ulceration of
Stomach..........Okra and apples
String beans and okra

To Cleanse
Uric Acid........Use a low-fat diet and take:

| | |
|---|---|
| asparagus | spinach |
| rhubarb | endive |
| cranberries | watercress |
| No flesh foods | |

Respiratory
Problems ........Violet leaves, chickweed

Staph ................Oxoquinidine (from the quinine tree)

Signs of Pancreas
Trouble ..........Sense of oppression in the stomach region.
Sensation as if a morsel were sticking in

the throat. Use iodine very diluted in 1
glass of water. (1 drop)

Sinus................Horseradish, onion, turnips, mustard, radishes

Strep................Cucumbers

When **Thyroid** is low, protein digestion is impaired

Tumor..............Eggplant peel and pulp, kelp

Osteoarthritis......Can be helped by feeding the pituitary
gland.

# VALUE OF FOODS

## For Good Health

For your convenience, I have arranged the value of different foods so you may easily find the variety you wish to eat.

Group I — Most healing
Group II — Supplement to Group I
Group III — Once in a while
Group IV — When you are in the prime of health and can afford to be fancy
Group V — Never

## Group I

| | | |
|---|---|---|
| Fresh fruit | Raw vegetables | Sprouted wheat |
| Fresh juices | Salads | Sprouted seeds |
| | Herbs | |
| | Raw juices | |
| Fresh milk, | Nuts | Oils: |
| (from healthy | Almonds | cold pressed |
| cows) | Sunflower seeds | Maple syrup |
| Yoghurt | Flax seeds | Date sugar |
| Kefir | Sesame Seeds | |

## Group II

Dried fruit
Fruit juices,
  in bottles

Milk,
  Pasteurized
Cheeses

Vegetables,
  cooked
Dried legumes

Eggs

Brown rice
Bread, whole
  wheat
Raw honey
Cereals, whole
  grain
Potatoes, boiled
  or baked in skins

## Group III

Fruit, when
  canned and
  sweetened

Skim milk
Cheeses,
  Pasteurized

Heated oil
Heated honey
Fish, chicken and
  turkey dishes

## Group IV

Fruit jellies
  and jams
Fruit pies

Boiled milk
Chocolate milk
Puddings

Vegetables,
  canned

Sausages
Fried meat

White bread
Noodles
White rice
White flour
Refined oils
Cheap margarine
Lard

## Group V

Sugar
Candies
Chocolate

Cakes
Cookies

Synthetic foods

# SUGAR STORY

Sugar is a very concentrated food. That means it has lots of calories and calories heat your body quickly. Imagine a coal stove. The harder the coal, the longer and more equal is the fire burning. In fact, it gleams all night. But when you put straw or paper in your stove, it burns a little while, makes lots of flames and is gone.

This is the way, when you feed your body heat with so much sugar, it makes energy very quickly, but after that, it leaves you exhausted and cranky. Cranky people are not very pleasant. The worst thing is crankiness. It is contagious and other people become cranky too, and then the world does not look so very sunny and beautiful any longer.

# SPROUTING

**Supplies Needed:** A container of any kind that has a lid, such as a canning jar. A piece of cheese cloth and a rubber band OR a piece of plastic screen and a two-piece canning lid.

**What To Sprout:** Any WHOLE nut, WHOLE grain or WHOLE seed that is untreated. (That is why I recommend purchasing them from a reliable source, such as an Organic Farmer, or from your local Health Food Store.)

**How To Sprout:** STERILIZE you container. It is best to keep using the same container over and over again, once you've started.

MEASURE your seeds according to the amounts you wish to use. I recommend these amounts for a one-quart container:

ALFALFA, 1 tbsp. sprouted 7 days

MUNG BEANS, 3 tbsp. sprouted 4 days

LENTILS, 6 tbsp. sprouted 4 days

FENUGREEK, 6 tbsp. sprouted 4 days

RINSE the seeds lightly before the next step, just as a precaution.

SOAK OVERNIGHT in three times more volume of water than the seeds, since they expand through the soaking process. Small seeds may be soaked from 6 to 8 hours, medium seeds from 8 to 10 hours and large seeds from 10 to 12 hours.

COVER the container with cheese cloth secured with a rubber band.

DRAIN THOROUGHLY after the correct length of soaking time.

DISTRIBUTE THE SEEDS gently around the sides of the jar.

PLACE ON AN ANGLE in the baking pan for better circulation of air. Put the bottom of the jar on the rim and the mouth of the jar in the pan. This will drain any excess moisture off the sprouts.

RINSE AS NEEDED.

REPEAT THE RINSING PROCESS for as many days as you wish your sprouts to grow.

TASTE your sprouts every day until they suit your taste buds. Remember with each passing day they get stronger in taste.

RESET ON THE ANGLE POSITION in the baking pan, for further draining between rinsings.

REFRIGERATE when they have reached their peak of unfoldment. Remove the cheese cloth and rubber band and put the top on the container to seal in the elements. This step will retard the growth of the sprouts, but please use them within a five-day period. They will last much longer than that, but they lose some of their nutritional content.

**Causes Of Mold:** Be sure the container has been sterilized. Put it in the hottest water possible with a little baking soda added for at least 20 minutes. Then wash regularly before use. Try to keep the temperature within a 68-72 degree zone. So keep them in a warm place in the winter and in the summer, a cool one.

Not draining thoroughly will also cause mold. Set in a large bowl at a 45 degree angle for about five minutes, after your quick draining. Then replace it at the above state angle.

**Place to Sprout:** Pick a spot that you frequently pass in your house each day. This will remind you to water them. Also you can observe and enjoy the marvelous process of life that is springing forth from the seeds.

**Time:** It just takes seconds to rinse them off, no more than putting a pot of water on the stove to boil. Your nutritional gain is phenomenal, and that alone makes it worth the extra effort of getting started.

# UNUSUAL HEALTH RECIPES
## Greek Yoghurt

3 quarts milk
1 cup heavy cream
5 tbsp. yoghurt
½ lemon (optional)

Heat cream and milk together, stir so it does not stick and cook 10 minutes. Remove from heat and cool only until comfortable to small finger (20 seconds).

Thin yoghurt in cup with part of milk, add lemon and remainder of milk, stir until blended.

Pour in large bowl or individual molds, cover well and keep in warm place 6 to 8 hours or overnight, until set. For thicker yoghurt, empty yoghurt into muslin bag and suspend to allow excess liquid to drain.

### Nut or Seed Milk

Blend well, first soaking:
1 cup nuts or seeds
1 cup cool water

Add:
2 tsp. honey
Sprinkle of sea salt
2 cups more water (or more) make as thick or thin
as you like.

Buzz again — chill.
Serve over fruit, cereals, or to drink.
Do the same with cashews; **almonds** are delicous, too.

## Poppyseed Milk

125 gr. poppyseed (or ½ cup)
4 cups milk (or water)

Grind the seed and soak for several hours.
Serve as an evening drink (excellent sleep remedy).

## Arthritis

On empty stomach:
1 tsp. soda
1 glass water

Repeat every hour, 3-4 times.
Also add ½ lb. soda to the bath tub. Soak for 15-20 minutes, 3 times a day for 5 weeks.

## Hormone Cereal

1 tbsp. sesame seeds
1 tbsp. sunflower seeds
1 tbsp. almonds
1 tbsp. chia seeds
1 tbsp. flax seeds
1 tbsp. raisins
apple juice

Grind seeds to a fine meal in the seed grinder or blender.
Place this mixture into a bowl.
Add raisins and enough apple juice to cover the seed mixture.
Allow to sit overnight. It is ready to eat in the morning as a cereal. Serves 2.

## Salad Rich in Potassium

1 part cabbage
1 part parsley
1 part carrots
1 part celery
Light oil-vinegar dressing with herbs

## Yoghurt

1 quart warm water
1⅓ cup non-instant dry milk
⅓ cup yoghurt

Mix milk and water in blender, add yoghurt, set in yoghurt dishes overnight.

## The Right Kind of Protein is Needed

Soak in pineapple juice overnight:
>⅜ cup sesame seed
>½ cup chia seed
>½ cup flax seed

Soak in prune juice:
>½ cup almonds
>½ cup filberts
>½ cup walnuts

Eat as is

## Canadian Health Salad

>1 small head cabbage, green
>1 bunch celery
>2-3 bell peppers
>1 handful carrots
>1 bunch fresh green onions
>2 bunches parsley

Grind all ingredients in a blender or food processor, so that the salad becomes compact, juicy and chewable—oil-vinegar dressing with herbs.

## Lentil or Wheat Sprout Patties

>4 cups lentil sprouts or wheat sprouts
>½ cup nut butter (peanut, almond, etc.)
>½ cup celery, finely chopped
>¼ cup onion, finely chopped
>1 or 2 small carrots, grated
>2 tsp. broth powder
>1 tsp. tamari soy sauce (optional)
>
>½ tsp. basil
>¼ tsp. sage

Grind sprouts and carrot by putting Through Champion juicer, using homegenizer attachment. Add other ingredients and mix well.

Form into patties. Place into greased baking pan. Broil if desired, for approximately 15-20 minutes. This may be served raw. Serves 5-6.

## Maple Baked Apple

>1 large apple
>butter
>pure maple syrup
>
>sun-dried raisins
>cinnamon

Core apple. Fill cavity with equal amounts of butter and maple syrup to which a few raisins and a dash of cinnamon have been added. Bake at 350 degrees for about 25 minutes. Serve hot. Serves 1.

# Onion Soup

**Vitamin C cannot be assimilated when PH is below 6.4.**

You have to prepare an onion soup (preparation time less than 10 minutes):

       1 lb. onion cut in small pieces

Cut with water and simer until done.

Add: 1 can mushroom soup and serve at once.

This will open the tissue so that Vitamin C is absorbed and utilized.


# Onion Soup with Fresh Mushrooms

Saute finely-cut onions in oil, butter and half and half.

Cut mushrooms in small pieces and add with water, salt and nutmeg.

Simmer and thicken lightly with unbleached flour or cornstarch or arrowroot starch.

Take from fire and add 1 tbsp. sour cream to each serving.

You can use yoghurt also.

People allergic to penicillin do poorly on mushroom.

You can also prepare:   eggplant-mushroom soup

                    vegetable-mushroom soup

                    rice, miso-mushroom soup

                    or any of the many varieties


# Eggplant Caviar

2 large eggplants (1 lb. size), halved lengthwise

1 large yellow onion, finely chopped

1 green pepper, seeded and finely chopped

3 tbsp. oil

2 tbsp. tomato paste

Juice of ½ lemon (2 tbsp.)

1 tsp. sugar

salt and pepper

Heat the oven to 325 degrees. Grease a baking pan large enough to hold the four eggplant halves. Place the eggplant face down, and bake them for 30 minutes. Peel off the skin, and finely chop the eggplant. Meanwhile, saute the onion and pepper in oil until they are soft and slightly browned. Add the eggplant, tomato paste, lemon juice and sugar. Fry the mixture for 10 minutes. Add salt and pepper to taste. Oversalt slightly, since the mixture will lose seasoning somewhat as it chills. Refrigerate the mixture in a glass or ceramic container. Serve it chilled, garnished with black olives and parsley sprigs. Serve it with triangles of pita bread or crackers as a spread or dip.

## Vegetable Broth

 2 quarts distilled water
 2 cups shredded celery
 2 cups shredded carrots
 2 tbsp. cut parsley
Bring to a full boil, cover and simmer for 20 minutes. Strain.
 Add:
 2 cups Tomato juice
 1 tsp. Vege-salt
 2 tsp. honey
Simmer again for 10 minutes.
Add your favorite sprouts just before serving.
This is a wonderful cleansing broth. Good anytime.
Variations made by adding onions, chives, beet tops, etc.

## Protein Drink

 2 cups carrot juice
 10 almonds
 2 tbsp. sunflower seeds, soaked
 1 tbsp. sesame seeds
 1 raw egg yolk
Blend for 2 minutes and add ice to chill.
 Add ½ cup sprouts

## For a Health Drink

 Take soaked lima beans, boil in plenty of water for 30 minutes. Drain the water off. Pour over peach tree leaves (1 tsp. per cup) and drink at least 2 cups a day.
 This drink is helpful against microscopic organisms.

## Vitality Drink

 1 pint milk
 2 tbsp. lecithin
 2 tbsp. Protesoy or any other high protein powder
 2 tsp. wheat germ oil
 2 egg yolks
 honey if wanted
This is for one day.

# Bircher-Musli

Take 3 tbsp. of rolled oats and soak over night in 1 cup water. The next morning add:

1 grated apple
1 tbsp. lemon juice
a few nuts
some cream

This is the basic recipe. The variation is endless. Instead of an apple, try fresh berries, pineapple, pears or banana. Always add a little lemon juice. Lemon juice is the adrenal stimulator and helps you face the day. Instead of cream, try milk, almond milk, sesame milk or soy milk. If you don't have fresh fruit, you can alsays soak raisins or dried fruit overnight. Add this to the Musli in the morning.

# Carrot Yoghurt Soup
### (Good hot or cold)

¼ cup butter or margarine
8 medium carrots scraped and sliced
3 medium onions, chopped
1 cup plain yoghurt
½ cup light cream
¼ cup chopped fresh chives, or
2 tbsp. freeze-dried chives

Melt butter or margarine in a large frying pan, saute carrot and onion until onion is tender. Add chicken broth or stock, cover and simmer for 1 hour.

Puree carrot and onion with liquid in blender. Transfer mixture to a 2-quart saucepan.

Add yoghurt and light cream, stirring until smooth.

Keep it on low heat until ready to serve, but do not allow to boil. Sprinkle with chives. This makes 7 cups, about 180 calories per cup serving.

# Eggplant Soup

3 cups diced eggplant
3 cups water
2 cups soybean milk
Dulse

Cut the eggplant into pieces and sprinkle with dulse. Let it sit for one hour. Press the juices out and cook in 3 cups of water until done. Add soybean milk and 1 tablespoon of butter or oil. Serve hot.

# Creamy Lettuce Soup

1 head lettuce
2 chicken bouillon cubes, crumbled
¾ cup water
2 tbsp. lemon juice
½ cup onion rings
¼ cup butter or margarine
¼ cup unbleached flour
2 cups milk
3 tbsp. water and 1 tbsp. lemon juice, blended

Core, rinse, and drain lettuce thoroughly; shred enough to measure 4 cups, packed. Chill any remaining lettuce in plastic bag or crisper for use at another time.

Combine shredded lettuce with bouillon cubes, water and lemon juice in blender; whir until smooth. Saute onion in butter in sauce pan until tender-crisp, but not browned; remove onion from pan with slotted spoon.

Blend flour into butter in pan; stir in milk. Cook, stirring, until mixture comes to boil and is thickened; blend in water-lemon juice-lettuce puree.

Add onion; heat through.

Serve at once with additional crisp shredded lettuce in center, if you wish. Serves 6.

## Sprout Drink

2 cups pineapple juice
1 cup sprouts (alfalfa, mung, etc.)
¼ banana
Slice of lemon (peeling and all, cut out of the
    middle section)

## Sprouted Breakfast Cereal

SOAK OVERNIGHT the sprouts that you want.
DRAIN AND RINSE the sprouts for two days.
USE per person:
    1 heaping teaspoon sunflower seeds
    1 heaping teaspoon pumpkin seeds
    1 heaping teaspoon sesame seeds

Use these sprouted seeds with your favorite cereal (cooked or cold) with yoghurt instead of milk. Fresh or frozen fruit may be added to cereal. For varieties, try:
    1 heaping teaspoon flax seed
    1 heaping teaspoon chia seed

Soak these seeds overnight, but use the next day with either fruit or cereal or with both.

119

## Sprouts Casserole

6 eggs
2 tablespoons salad oil
1 cup chopped parsley
2 large onions, chopped (about 1 cup)
2 cups cooked rice
2 cups sprouts
3 cups grated cheese
2 cups soy milk
2 tablespoons soy sauce

Save half the cheese for topping. Whip eggs and slowly fold in the other ingredients. Top with cheese. Bake 45 minutes at 350 degrees.


## Energy Drink

3 cups pineapple juice
1 cup water (distilled or spring)
1 cup alfalfa sprouts
½ cup comfrey leaves (3 or 4)
10 almonds


## A Wonderful Recipe for a Truly Natural Soft Drink

1 or 2 tbsp. Black Cherry Concentrate
to an 8 ounce glass of water (distilled preferably)
a few drops fresh lemon juice (optional)
Refreshing without the fizz!

Even bottling it in a huge "pop" bottle in the refrigerator, if it takes this kind of "window dressing" to make the transition from the Cola Addiction to a healthful drink. Since caffeine and sugar give a false lift, a chunk of cheese with the Cherry Pop offsets the LOW!


## Smart Sandwich

1 slice 7 grain bread
Butter well (or substitute mayonnaise) sprinkle generously with sage, few drops of lemon juice; add dulse (or a couple of Kelp Tablets)— slice in half, wrap in romaine lettuce leaves.

We urge that parents consult the nutritionally aware pediatrician or a capable nutritionist to investigate supplementation for improvement, especially in the area of mental acumen.

# Zucchini Bread

(Thanks to Mrs. Otto Kreft, Box 223, Vesta, Minn. 56292)

3 eggs (beat until foamy)
1⅓ cups sugar (natural)
⅓ cup honey
1 cup oil
1 tsp. cinnamon
dash nutmeg
1 tsp. salt
1 tsp. soda
¼ tsp. baking powder
1 tsp. vanilla
2 cups grated, unpeeled zucchini
3 cups unbleached flour
1 cup chopped nuts

Bake 35 minutes at 350° or until done.

# For Popsicle People

Try 1 tsp. Black Cherry Concentrate with water, per popsicle, when making your own, and avoid the synthetics here also.

**Great Breakfast for Everyone** from the "pokey" child to

## To restore balance in the unbalanced diet:

6 oz. tomato juice
3 tsp. liquid amino acid
½ tsp. Vitamin C granules
2 tsp. lecithin granules
1 tsp. wheat germ oil

Mix it well, preferably by shaking in a tightly covered jar, rather than a blender. To be taken 3 times daily.

# Books By Hanna Kroeger

**AGELESS REMEDIES FROM MOTHER'S KITCHEN** — You will laugh and be amazed at what all you can do in your own pharmacy, the kitchen. A rediscovered collection of time tested remedies for common complaints, using food and herbs often found in the kitchen. Over 700 recipes. $3.50

**ALLERGY BAKING RECIPES** — Easy recipes, tasty and tested for cookies, cakes, muffins, pancakes, breads, and pie crusts made without wheat; some without milk, eggs or yeast and using cereal free baking powder. $1.45

**ARTERIOSCLEROSIS** — Hanna's book explaining how and where arteriosclerosis can affect us and what to do about it. $1.00

**COOKBOOK FOR ELECTRO-CHEMICAL ENERGIES** — A unique cookbook designed to help you create and release electro-chemical energies through your diet. Over 300 recipes. $3.00

**GOD HELPS THOSE WHO HELP THEMSELVES** — Hanna's most complete book on natural healing helps us to understand the problems we may have on the physical, mental and spiritual planes. $6.95

**GOOD HEALTH THROUGH SPECIAL DIETS** — This book shows detailed outlines of different diets for different needs. Includes many natural ways to cleanse and strengthen the organs and bodily functions. $3.95

**INSTANT HERBAL LOCATOR** — A recently revised collection of Hanna's most effective herbal recipes in an easy to use cross reference guide. $3.50

**INSTANT VITAMIN-MINERAL LOCATOR** — A compact and comprehensive "How-To" vitamin and mineral gude. Shows nutritive value of vitamins and minerals and what symptoms they work for. $2.25

**MAGNETO THERAPY** — The laying on of hands, a time proven, very effective method to reestablish the electromagnetic energies of your body. $1.50

**OLD TIME REMEDIES** — A dynamic collection of natural remedies from Eastern and Western cultures. There are 20 fast-cleansing methods and many ways to rebuild your health. Essential to a better understanding of improving your health and the vitality of your organs. $3.50

**RECIPES FOR A CANCER-FREE LIFESTYLE** — An excellent guide to help strengthen the body in this age old fight. Recipes from around the world. Physical and Spiritual food to reinforce the body's natural defenses against cancer. $2.95

**THE PENDULUM, THE BIBLE AND YOUR SURVIVAL** — Explains one method of acquiring your sixth sense, your intuition. A must to help your families achieve better health in today's stressful environment. $1.50

**THE SEVEN SPIRITUAL CAUSES OF ILL HEALTH** — An informative guide that goes beyond the physical and into the spiritual aspects of our health. $7.00

---

## ORDERING INFORMATION

To purchase any of the products listed in this catalog contact your local health food store or call or write:

New Age Foods
1122 Pearl St.
Boulder, CO 80302
(303) 443-0755